总主编 房敏
主编 林乾程 王乾炤 朱清广

中医传统锻炼

六字诀

Traditional Chinese Medicine Exercise
Liuzijue (Chinese-English)

汉英双语

中国教育出版传媒集团
高等教育出版社·北京

内容简介

本书为中国传统医药国际交流丛书之一。六字诀是一种独特的传统锻炼方法，研习者通过吐纳呼吸和动作配合，可以达到强身健体、调节身心的目的。

本书有五章，分别介绍了六字诀的源流、理论基础、锻炼特点、锻炼要领，以及常见病的防治。全书采用英汉对照的形式，并配有图片，语言通俗易懂，动作分解详细，方便国内外读者研习。

图书在版编目（CIP）数据

六字诀：汉、英 / 林乾炪，王程，朱清广主编. — 北京：高等教育出版社，2025.5. — (中医传统锻炼 / 房敏总主编). — ISBN 978-7-04-064651-1

Ⅰ. R214

中国国家版本馆 CIP 数据核字第 20255B79W8 号

ZHONGYI CHUANTONG DUANLIAN: LIUZIJUE (HAN-YING SHUANGYU)

| 策划编辑 | 龙 杰 | 责任编辑 | 王 羽 | 封面设计 | 王 琰 | 版式设计 | 杨 树 |
| 责任绘图 | 黄云燕 | 责任校对 | 高 歌 | 责任印制 | 存 怡 |

出版发行	高等教育出版社	网　　址	http://www.hep.edu.cn
社　　址	北京市西城区德外大街4号		http://www.hep.com.cn
邮政编码	100120	网上订购	http://www.hepmall.com.cn
印　　刷	肥城新华印刷有限公司		http://www.hepmall.com
开　　本	880mm×1230mm　1/32		http://www.hepmall.cn
印　　张	5.125		
字　　数	150 千字	版　　次	2025 年 5 月第 1 版
购书热线	010-58581118	印　　次	2025 年 5 月第 1 次印刷
咨询电话	400-810-0598	定　　价	49.00 元

本书如有缺页、倒页、脱页等质量问题，请到所购图书销售部门联系调换
版权所有　侵权必究
物料号　64651-00

编写委员会

总主编

房　敏

主　编

林乾炤　　王　程　　朱清广

副主编

孙武权　　郭光昕　　姚重界

程艳彬　　黄思彭　　摆　雪

Editorial Committee

Editor-in-Chief

Fang Min

Chief Editors

Lin Qianzhao　　Wang Cheng　　Zhu Qingguang

Associate Editors

Sun Wuquan　　Guo Guangxin　　Yao Chongjie

Cheng Yanbin　　Huang Sipeng　　Bai Xue

总序

中医传统锻炼，作为中医非药物疗法的重要组成部分，历经千年传承与实践，被广泛认可为既防治疾病又强身健体的有效方法，其中深藏着中医文化的深厚底蕴与无尽智慧。这些锻炼功法包括八段锦、六字诀、少林内功、太极拳、五禽戏、易筋经等，它们强调个体的自我身心调节和自我治愈能力，通过调形、调息、调神引导身体内在的能量来平衡和修复身体的机能，从而达到防治疾病和提高健康水平的目的。

由来自上海中医药大学和新疆医科大学的作者团队联合组织编写的中医传统锻炼系列图书包括以上六种功法，不仅向读者介绍了传统功法的原理、历史，更创新性地将这些古老的智慧与目前慢性病的防治相融合，使传统功法在现代社会焕发新生。每一种图书都深入剖析了一种特定的功法，并提供了清晰易懂的操作指南与研习建议，使读者能够根据自己的健康状况、兴趣爱好及时间安排进行个性化调整，制订专属的健康计划。通过进行中医传统锻炼，不仅可以有效降低慢性疾病的发病率和患病率，还能显著提高健康素养，促进心理健康，全面提升整体健康水平。让我们共同走进这套图书，探寻中医传统锻炼的魅力，传承并弘扬中华优秀传统文化，让古老功法在新时代焕发出更加耀眼的光芒！

编者
2024 年 8 月

Introduction

Traditional Chinese Medicine (TCM) exercises, as an important part of non-pharmacological therapies in Chinese medicine, have been passed down and practiced for thousands of years, and are widely recognized as an effective method for both preventing and curing diseases and strengthening the body, which is deeply embedded in the profound heritage and endless wisdom of Chinese medicine culture. These exercise techniques include Baduanjin, Liuzijue, Shaolin Neigong, Taijiquan, Wuqinxi, Yijinjing, etc. They emphasize the individual's ability to regulate the body and mind and self-heal, and they guide the body's inner energy to balance and repair the body's functions by regulating the form, breath and spirit, thus achieving the purpose of treating diseases and improving health.

The Traditional Chinese Medicine exercise series books, which include the above six exercise methods, are jointly organized and written by a team of authors from the Shanghai University of Traditional Chinese Medicine and Xinjiang Medical University. These books not only introduce the principles and history of the traditional Chinese medicine exercises, but also innovatively integrate these ancient wisdoms with the current prevention and treatment of chronic diseases, revitalizing traditional exercise methods in the modern world. Each book provides an in-depth analysis of a specific exercise method, as well as clear and easy-to-follow instructions and study suggestions, enabling readers to make personalized adjustments to their own health conditions, interests, and schedules, and to develop an exclusive health plan. By practicing traditional Chinese medicine exercises, not only can we effectively reduce the incidence and prevalence of chronic diseases, but also significantly enhance health literacy, promote mental health, and improve overall health. Let's walk into this set of books together, explore the charm of traditional Chinese medicine exercises, inherit and carry forward the excellent traditional Chinese culture, and let the ancient exercises in the new era shine more brightly!

Editor
August 2024

前言

在中华悠久的历史文化中，传统锻炼方法占据有重要地位。六字诀，作为一种独特而古老的健身方法，深受历代养生家和武术家的推崇。

六字诀最早见于南北朝时期陶弘景所著《养性延命录》，传至唐代名医孙思邈，按五行相生之顺序，配合四时之季节进一步完善，奠定了六字诀治病之基础。

中医传统锻炼方法众多，各具特点，研习者须知学无止境，应虚心求教，以博采众长，为发扬中华传统医学文化而努力。最后提醒各位读者，本功法锻炼主要是为慢性病的防治提供重要参考，有健康问题时首选就医诊疗。

本书配有视频，读者扫描二维码输入20位防伪码（刮开涂层可见）可观看视频。

编者
2024 年 8 月

Foreword

In the long history and culture of China, traditional exercise methods occupy an important position. The Liuzijue of Traditional Chinese Medicine Exercise, as a unique and ancient fitness method, has been highly esteemed by health cultivators and martial artists throughout the ages.

The Liuzijue was first recorded in the *The Record of Naturing Life and Prolonging Life* by Tao Hongjing during the Northern- Southern Dynasties. The Liuzijue for Healing was further perfected by the famous Tang Dynasty physician Sun Simiao, who arranged it according to the sequence of the Five Elements and coordinated it with the four seasons of the year. This laid the foundation for the Liuzijue for healing.

Traditional Chinese Medicine Exercise offers a variety of exercise methods, each with its own unique characteristics. Readers need to know that learning is endless, and should be humble in seeking advice to acquire the best from others, striving to promote the culture of traditional Chinese medicine. Finally, I would like to remind all our readers that the practice of this exercise method is primarily intended to provide an important reference for the prevention and treatment of chronic diseases, and for health issues, medical diagnosis and treatment should be the first choice.

The book includes supplementary videos. You can scan the QR code and enter the 20-digit security code (visible after scratching of the coating) to access the video content.

Editor
August 2024

目录

第一章　六字诀的源流

第二章　六字诀的基础理论

第一节　阴阳学说 …………………………………………14
第二节　经络学说 …………………………………………16
第三节　气血学说 …………………………………………18
第四节　人体运动学 ………………………………………19

第三章　六字诀的特点

第一节　平衡阴阳 …………………………………………24
第二节　内敛精神 …………………………………………27
第三节　调整呼吸 …………………………………………29
第四节　变易筋骨 …………………………………………31

第四章　六字诀分步解析

预备式 ………………………………………………………36
第一式　"嘘"字诀 …………………………………………37

Contents

Chapter 1 The Origins and Development of Liuzijue

Chapter 2 The Theoretical Foundations of Liuzijue

Section 1 The Yin-Yang Theory ···14
Section 2 The Meridian Theory ···16
Section 3 The Theory of Qi and Blood ·····································18
Section 4 Human Kinesiology ···19

Chapter 3 Characteristics of Liuzijue

Section 1 Balancing Yin and Yang ···24
Section 2 Cultivating Inner Spirit ···27
Section 3 Adjusting Breathing ··29
Section 4 Transforming Muscles and Bones ······························31

Chapter 4 Step-by-Step Analysis of Liuzijue

Preparatory Posture ··36
  One "Xu" Zijue ··37

第二式	"呵"字诀	40
第三式	"呼"字诀	44
第四式	"呬"字诀	47
第五式	"吹"字诀	51
第六式	"嘻"字诀	55
收势		60

第五章　常见病的防治

第一节	慢性阻塞性肺疾病	64
第二节	支气管哮喘	68
第三节	咳嗽	72
第四节	胸闷	76
第五节	心悸	79
第六节	颈椎病	82
第七节	腰痛	93
第八节	肾虚	103
第九节	胃肠功能紊乱	107
第十节	骨质疏松症	110
第十一节	脂肪肝	113
第十二节	膝痛	117
第十三节	肩痛	123
第十四节	头痛	129
第十五节	慢性疲劳综合征	133
第十六节	便秘	136
第十七节	肺结节	139
第十八节	焦虑	142

参 考 文 献

Two	"He" Zijue	40
Three	"Hu" Zijue	44
Four	"Si" Zijue	47
Five	"Chui" Zijue	51
Six	"Xi" Zijue	55
Closing Posture		60

Chapter 5 Prevention and Treatment of Common Diseases

Section 1	Chronic Obstructive Pulmonary Disease	64
Section 2	Bronchial Asthma	68
Section 3	Cough	72
Section 4	Chest Tightness	76
Section 5	Palpitations	79
Section 6	Cervical Spondylosis	82
Section 7	Lower Back Pain	93
Section 8	Kidney Deficiency	103
Section 9	Gastrointestinal Dysfunction	107
Section 10	Osteoporosis	110
Section 11	Fatty Liver	113
Section 12	Knee Pain	117
Section 13	Shoulder Pain	123
Section 14	Headache	129
Section 15	Chronic Fatigue Syndrome	133
Section 16	Constipation	136
Section 17	Pulmonary Nodules	139
Section 18	Anxiety	142

第一章 六字诀的源流

六字诀是我国古代流传下来的一种将呼吸吐纳与形体动作相结合的养生功法，是在中国传统文化理论、中医学理论和导引功法的指导下发展而来的长息吐气之法。此功法是以"嘘、呵、呼、呬、吹、嘻"六字，分别对应肝、心、脾、肺、肾、三焦等脏腑经络，结合动作导引，再与四季相对应，以达到调节全身气息的作用。

六字诀需要长期习练、循序渐进、反复体会，通过呼吸、形体和意念的锻炼，专注"意、气、力"，有利于调节人们的"精、气、神"，促进人类的心理健康及形体健康，达到调神和强身的统一。

古人早已认识到，通过调息调身锻炼，可祛病强身、延年益寿，道出了吐纳功法的奥秘。六字诀最早记载于南北朝陶弘景的《养性延命录》。此后，历代医家也均有对六字诀的论述，尤其在六字诀的方法理论及应用上有不少的发展与补充。经过历代人不断发展和完善的六字诀理论、方法和应用，虽与陶弘景在书中记载的古法有所不同，但其养生、防治疾病的功用逐渐得到认可。到了现代，人们更加重视未病先防的理念，提出功法锻炼是疾病预防的重要方法之一，掀起了动功锻炼的热潮。六字诀进一步得到了规范化管理和科学推广，作者在传统六字气诀功法的基础上改良创作了健身运动六字诀，以满足全民养生运动的需要。

Chapter 1　The Origins and Development of Liuzijue

The Liuzijue is a traditional health-preserving exercise method passed down from ancient China, which combines breathing techniques with physical movements. Developed under the guidance of traditional Chinese cultural and medical theories, as well as guiding exercise methods, it involves long exhalation and inhalation techniques. This method utilizes the six sounds "Xu, He, Hu, Si, Chui, Xi" to correspond to the liver, heart, spleen, lungs, kidneys, and triple energizer respectively. Combined with specific movements and synchronized with the four seasons, it aims to regulate the body's overall energy flow.

The practice of Liuzijue requires long-term, progressive, and repeated training. Through the exercises of breathing, physical movements, and mental focus, practitioners concentrate on "intention, breath, and strength." This practice is beneficial for regulating one's "essence, energy, and spirit," promoting both mental and physical health, and achieving harmony between mind and body for spiritual and physical well-being.

Ancient scholars long ago recognized breath regulation and physical exercises contributed to dispelling illness, strengthening the body, and prolonging life, revealing the secrets of breathing exercises. The earliest records of the Liuzijue can be found in Tao Hongjing's *The Record of Nurturing Life and Prolonging Life* during the Northern and Southern Dynasties. Subsequently, generations of physicians have discussed the Liuzijue, with considerable development and supplementation, particularly in its theory, methods and applications. Through continuous development and refinement by successive generations, albeit the differences from the ancient methods recorded by Tao Hongjing, the health-preserving and disease-preventing functions of the Liuzijue gradually gained recognition. In modern times, there is a greater emphasis on the concept of preventive healthcare. It is proposed that exercise methods are one of the important methods for disease prevention, leading to a surge in the popularity of exercise training. The Liuzijue has further been standardized and scientifically promoted. Based on traditional Six-Character Qigong methods, fitness-oriented Liuzijue has been innovated to meet the needs of nationwide fitness movements.

1. 南北朝时期

"六字气诀"功法最早记载于距今 1 500 多年前南北朝时期梁代陶弘景的《养性延命录》一书。距今 5 000 多年前的新石器时代马家窑文化时期的出土文物彩陶罐的人形浮雕，这尊人像呈现出张口呼吸吐纳的站桩练功姿势，说明古人已经懂得运用呼吸吐纳，通过调息调身练功来调和阴阳、延年益寿。《黄帝内经》等一系列的文献也说明了我们的先人对呼吸吐纳养生意义有了更具体的认识。《庄子·刻意》记述："吹呴呼吸，吐故纳新，熊经鸟伸，为寿而已矣。"道出了呼吸吐纳之术，也指出了当时学习模仿动物动作，作为"养形之道"，养生之法。再到后来的东晋时期，葛洪所著的《神仙传》指出："士大夫学道者多矣，然所谓八段锦、六字气，特导引吐纳而已。"也说明我们的先人逐渐掌握了呼吸吐纳法。

1. Northern and Southern Dynasties period

During the Northern and Southern Dynasties, over 1 500 years ago, Tao Hongjing of the Liang Dynasty first recorded the Liuzijue in his book *The Record of Nurturing Life and Prolonging Life*. The figurines on unearthed colored pottery jars dating back over 5 000 years to the Majiayao culture of the Neolithic Age depict a standing posture of breathing exercises, indicating that ancient people understood the use of breath regulation for harmonizing Yin and Yang and prolonging life. Subsequent documents such as *Huangdi's Classic on Medicine* further illustrate our ancestors' more specific understanding of the health benefits of breath regulation. Zhuangzi's "Deliberate Effort" records: "Blowing and exhaling breath, expelling the old and taking in the new, stretching like a bear and extending like a bird, are practices for longevity." It elucidates the technique of breath regulation and also points out the learning of imitating animal movements at that time, as a way of "nurturing form" and preserving health. By the Eastern Jin Dynasty, Ge Hong's *Biographies of the Divine Immortals* pointed out: "There are many scholars learning the Tao, but the so-called Eight Section Brocade and Six-Character Qigong are just about guiding breath regulation." This indicates that our ancestors gradually mastered the technique of breath regulation.

During the Wei, Jin, Northern and Southern Dynasties, Tao Hongjing, as a Taoist and physician, based on the theoretical foundation of previous Qigong and health-preservation practices, compiled The *Record of Nurturing Life and Prolonging Life* with a more detailed description of the methods of breath regulation and "vocalizing the breath". It states: "In all forms of Qigong, one inhales through the nose and exhales through the mouth. This practice, done gently, is called long breathing. There is one type of inhalation and six types of exhalation. The single inhalation is called Xi, while the six types of exhalation Chui, Hu, Xi, He, Xu, Si, are all methods of long exhalation." His proposal of using breath to treat illnesses and the techniques of guiding massage were widely loved and highly accepted, and were learned and inherited.

2. During the Sui and the Tang Dynasties

During the Sui and the Tang Dynasties, it was a golden age for the development of exercise methods. In the Sui Dynasty, Chao Yuanfang's *Discourse on the Origin and Symptoms of Various Diseases* proposed principles for differentiating and applying massage techniques, making breath regulation an important part of guiding

引效果。呼吸吐纳可以调息调神，肢体动作具有养形的作用。隋代佛教天台宗创始人智顗将六字诀的吐纳养身法用于佛学坐禅止观法门。唐代药王孙思邈首创"大呼细呼、大吹细吹、大嘘细嘘、大呵细呵、大唏细唏、大呬细呬"之法，指出皆须左右导引三百六十遍，无有不瘥也。他强调吐气如声，而非发出声音，与陶弘景提倡的"气声逐字"，有所不同。至此，药王孙思邈以后大多数皆以"耳不得闻其声"的修炼方法。他重视调气之法作为治病和养生功法，主张导引术与六字诀相结合。晚唐医家、道家胡愔改变了六字与五脏的配属，改肺"嘘"为肺"呬"，改心"呼"为心"呵"，改肝"呵"为肝"嘘"，改脾"唏"为脾"呼"，改肾"呬"为肾"吹"，另增胆"嘻"之法。

methods. He emphasized that breath regulation, combined with physical movements and mental focus, could enhance the effectiveness of guidance. Breath regulation can regulate the mind and body, while physical movements contribute to nurturing the body. In the Sui Dynasty, Zhiyi, the founder of the Tiantai School of Buddhism, used the breath regulation method of Liuzijue in the practice of Buddhist meditation. In the Tang Dynasty, the medical sage Sun Simiao's pioneered the method of "loud exhalation and soft exhalation, loud blowing and soft blowing, loud hissing and soft hissing, loud sighing and soft sighing, loud panting and soft panting", emphasizing the need to guide the breath three hundred and sixty times in each direction, which would lead to complete recovery. He emphasized that exhalation should be like a sound but not actually produce a sound, which differed from Tao Hongjing's advocacy of "vocalizing the breath". Subsequently, most practitioners followed the method of "practicing without producing sound". He attached great importance to the method of regulating Qi as a method for treating diseases and preserving health, advocating the combination of guiding techniques with Liuzijue. Later in the late Tang Dynasty, the medical and Taoist practitioner Hu Yin changed the allocation of the Six Characters to the Five Internal Organs, replacing lung "Xu" with lung "Si", heart "Hu" with heart "He", liver "He" with liver "Xu", spleen "Xi" with spleen "Hu", kidney "Si" with kidney "Chui", and additionally introduced the method of gallbladder "Xi".

3. The Song, Yuan, Ming, and Qing dynasties

During the Song Dynasty, Zou Pu'an's *TaiShang YuZhou LiuZi QiJue* provides the most detailed exposition of the theory and methods of Liuzijue. He proposed specific requirements for pronunciation and breathing during the practice of Liuzijue, affirming the necessity of making sounds while exhaling, emphasizing the volume of sound heard by one's own ears as the measure. He believed that only by vocalizing could one distinguish the notes of Gong, Shang, Jiao, Zhi, and Yu, coordinate with the five viscera, vibrate the five viscera, and achieve better results, which he referred to as "wind breathing." Additionally, he included preparatory exercises such as tooth tapping, stirring the sea, and swallowing saliva. In his discourse, not only did the attribution of viscera change, but the sequence of exercises also correspondingly changed, showing a trend from mutual restraint to mutual generation. Among them, only between "Si" and "Xu" is there still mutual restraint, starting from the heart Fire of the Five Elements, with the

3. 宋元明清时期

宋代邹朴庵的《太上玉轴六字气诀》最为详细地论述了六字诀的理论与方法，提出了对于六字诀锻炼时的读音方法和呼吸的具体要求，肯定了吐字时需要发出声音，强调以自己耳朵听到的声量为度，认为只有发声才能区分宫、商、角、徵、羽，才能配合五脏，能振动五脏，才有更好的效果，并称其为"风呼吸"。而且还加了叩齿、搅海、咽津等预备功。他的论述中不仅脏腑归属发生变化，其练习的顺序也相应变化，呈现由相克向相生变化的趋势。其中，只有"呬""嘘"之间还是相克，而且仍起于五行之心火，取先泄心之火毒的意思。

金元四大家的刘完素，提出将六字气诀与五行学说相结合。明代冷谦将六字诀与四季结合了起来，提出按季节练习各字诀的简单易行的养生方法，明确说明了六字气诀功法与季节的关联性，肯定了六字诀是一种可驱邪扶正、延年益寿的呼吸吐纳法。在其治疗机理方面，明代龚居中指出："呵则通于心，去心家一切热气；嘘则通于肝，去肝经一切热聚之气；吹则通于肾，去肾中一切虚热之气；呬则通于肺，去肺家一切积气；呼则通于脾，去脾家一切浊气；嘻则通于胆，去胆中一切客热之气"。

后来的文献在六字与脏腑的对应归属上，大体都沿用了宋代邹朴庵的论述，只是将胆（嘻）改为三焦（嘻），因为后人认

intention of First draining the Fire poison of the heart.

Liu Wansu, one of the four great masters of the Jin and Yuan dynasties proposed combining Liuzijue with the theory of the Five Elements. In the Ming Dynasty, Leng Qian combined Liuzijue with the four seasons, proposing a simple and practical method of health preservation by practicing each word according to the season. He explicitly stated the correlation between the method of Liuzijue and the seasons, affirming that Liuzijue is a breathing technique that can expel evils, support righteousness, and prolong life. Regarding its therapeutic mechanism, Gong Juzhong of the Ming Dynasty pointed out: "'He' connects with the heart, eliminating heart-related heat; 'Xu' connects with the liver, eliminating all heat accumulation in the liver meridian; 'Chui' connects with the kidney, eliminating all empty heat in the kidney; 'Si' connects with the lungs, eliminating all accumulated Qi in the lungs; 'Hu' connects with the spleen, eliminating all turbid Qi in the spleen; 'Xi' connects with the gallbladder, eliminating all heat caused by cold in the gallbladder."

The later literature on the correspondence between the six syllables and the visera organs mostly follows the discourse of Zou Pu'an from the Song Dynasty, except that the gallbladder (Xi) has been changed to triple energizer (Xi). This is because later generations believed that "Xi" connects to the Shaoyang meridian, which can regulate the gallbladder meridian as well as the triple energizer meridian. In traditional Chinese medicine, "triple energizer governs the pivot", and regulating triple energizer can harmonize the body's Qi circulation. The function of the triple energizer is precisely to facilitate the circulation of Qi throughout the body.

After the Ming and Qing Dynasties, a unified Chinese phonetic annotation method emerged. Recorded in *HeLuo JingYun* by Jiang Shenxiu during the Qing Dynasty: "Human speech emanates from the throat, passes through the tongue, and touches the teeth, incisors, and lips, corresponding to the Five Elements. Throat sound corresponds to Earth, tongue sound to Fire, tooth sound to Wood, incisor sound to Metal, and lip sound to Water." This formed the correspondence between the Five Elements, five sounds, and five visera. Through the refinement and innovation of numerous physicians and Qigong practitioners throughout the ages, the Liuzijue gradually evolved to be practiced in accordance with the seasonal cycle and the generation sequence of the Five Elements. This further accumulated a wealth of theoretical guidance and techniques. The mechanism of disease prevention and treatment in Liuzijue was

为"嘻"通少阳经脉，既可疏通胆经，又可疏通三焦经脉。中医认为"少阳为枢"，通少阳即可调理全身气机，三焦的作用正是通行全身诸气。

明清以后，有了统一的汉字注音方法。清代江慎修所著《河洛精蕴》中记载："人之言出于喉，掉于舌，触击于牙、齿、唇，以应五行。喉音为土，舌音为火，牙音为木，齿音为金，唇音为水。"形成了五行五音五脏的对应关系。经过历代大量的医家、练功家提炼更新之后，六字诀基本按四季循环、五行相生顺序练习，进一步积累了大量的导引、功法的理论，六字诀的防治疾病机理得到了进一步系统和规范的整理，辅以肢体动作将吐纳与导引结合起来，形成了独特的锻炼风格。

4. 现代的继承和发展

国家体育总局健身气功管理中心组织专家将各门各派的六字诀进行梳理，重新编排，坚持以传统六字诀继承为主导，在不同版本传统六字诀基础上，编撰一套适合现代人生活和工作方式的健身气功。"六字诀"功法是呼吸法训练结合了肢体的运动，具有加强肢体的运动力量和承受能力以形引气、以气导形作用。每个字诀的正确发音，配合动作导引，来调整和控制体内气息的升降出入，肝嘘、心呵、脾呼、肺呬、肾吹、三焦嘻等方法，增强呼吸吐纳的功效。每个动作简单、优美，便于大众记忆、习练，是人们强身健体、防治疾病的常练功法。

further systematically and normatively organized. Coupled with bodily movements that combine breathing and guidance, it formed a unique style of exercise.

4. The inheritance and development in modern times

Health Qigong Management Center under the General Administration of Sport of China has organized experts to sort out and rearrange the Liuzijue from various schools and sects, adhering to the traditional inheritance of Liuzijue as the main principle. Based on different versions of the traditional Liuzijue, they have compiled a set of Qigong exercises suitable for modern lifestyles and work patterns. The Liuzijue method combines breathing techniques with bodily movements, aiming to strengthen the body's physical strength and resilience by guiding Qi with form and shaping form with Qi. Each syllable is pronounced correctly, accompanied by movement guidance, to adjust and control the ascent and descent of Qi within the body. Methods such as liver exhaling, heart inhaling, spleen exhaling, lung hissing, kidney blowing, and triple energizer exhaling enhance the effectiveness of breath regulation. Each movement is simple and graceful, easy to remember and practice, making it a common exercise method for strengthening the body, maintaining health, and preventing and treating diseases.

第二章 六字大明陀罗尼

第二章 六字诀的基础理论

Chapter 2 The Theoretical Foundations of Liuzijue

第一节 阴阳学说
Section 1　The Yin-Yang Theory

六字诀在长期的医疗实践发展和形成过程中受到了阴阳学说的影响。在六字诀呼吸吐纳方面，呼气发声吐字的时候属阳，吸气气沉丹田的时候属阴；在六字诀动作导引上，动作向上、向外展开的为阳，可以提升阳气；向下、向里内收的为阴，可以滋阴潜阳。

阴阳学说是我国古代哲学家们创立的朴素的对立统一理论，是古代哲学的唯物论和辩证法。阴阳是代表事物和现象互相对立而又互相统一的两面，包含对立制约、互根互用的两方面，始终处于运动变化和相互作用的状态。古代医学家们将阴阳概念应用于中医学理论之中，用于观察分析人体生理、病理等现象，解决疾病的治疗、预防问题，阐释了

In the process of long-term medical practice and development, Liuzijue was influenced by the theory of Yin and Yang. Regarding the breathing and exhalation in Liuzijue, exhaling while vocalizing is considered Yang, while inhaling and sinking the Qi to the Dantian is considered Yin. In terms of the movement guidance in Liuzijue, movements that expand upwards or outwards are considered Yang, which can enhance Yang Qi; movements that contract downwards or inwards are considered Yin, which can nourish Yin and subdue Yang.

The theory of Yin and Yang was established by ancient Chinese philosophers as a primitive theory of opposition and unity, representing the materialism and dialectics of ancient philosophy. Yin and Yang represent the two sides of things and phenomena that are mutually opposed yet unified, encompassing aspects of opposition, constraint, mutual dependence, and mutual utilization, always in a state of motion, change, and interaction. Ancient medical practitioners, by applying the concept of Yin and Yang to the theories of traditional Chinese medicine, observed and analyzed phenomena in human physiology and pathology, addressed issues of disease treatment and prevention. They elucidated the basic laws of human life activities and the relationship between humans and the natural world and emphasized a holistic view of "unity between heaven and man". Gradually, they developed the foundation of the theoretical system of traditional Chinese medicine based on the theory of Yin and Yang to guide clinical medical practice.

Ancient people used Yin and Yang to classify all things and phenomena in the natural world, categorizing bright, warm, and active attributes as Yang; and dark, cold, and static attributes as Yin. Similarly, for the human body, substances and phenomena with functions such as propulsion, elevation, warmth, and stimulation are considered Yang, while those with functions such as consolidation, settling, coolness, and inhibition are considered Yin. *The Book of Changes* states: "Establishing the principles of heaven, it is called Yin and Yang," which philosophically summarizes the basic laws of the generation, development, and changes of things. *Hangdi's Classic on Medicine* states: "The life of a person has form, which cannot be separated from Yin and Yang," explaining that the human body itself embodies a relationship of mutual opposition and interdependence, including the body's

人体生命活动的基本规律及人与自然界的关系，强调"天人合一"的整体观，逐渐发展出以阴阳学说为基础的中医学理论体系，指导医学临床实践。

古人用阴与阳划分自然界一切事物和现象，将明亮、温暖、运动的属阳；晦暗、寒冷、静止的属阴。同样，对于人体来说，具有推动、升举、温煦、兴奋等作用的物质及现象为阳，具有凝聚、沉降、凉润、抑制等作用的物质及现象为阴。《周易》指出："立天之道，曰阴与阳"，从哲学高度概括了阴阳乃事物发生发展变化的基本规律。《黄帝内经》曰："人生有形，不离阴阳"，说明了人体本身是相互对立、相互依存的对立统一关系，包含了人体组织、器官、脏腑及经络。"天地之道，以阴阳二气而造化万物；人生之理，以阴阳二气长养百骸"，指出了阴阳的对立统一、协调平衡维系着人体的生命进程。

tissues, organs, viscera, and meridians. "The Tao of heaven and earth creates all things with the two Qi of Yin and Yang; the principle of human life nurtures the hundred bones with the two Qi of Yin and Yang," indicating that the opposition, unity, coordination, and balance of Yin and Yang maintain the life processes of the human body.

第二节　经络学说
Section 2　The Meridian Theory

古人以砭刺、导引、推拿、气功等方法进行治疗或保健，且依据当时的解剖知识观察生理和病理状态下的经络感传现象，在长期医疗实践中反复观察和归纳总结经络理论知识，从而形成了经络学说。它是在阴阳五行学说指导下发展起来的，是中医学理论体系的重要组成部分，包含人体经络系统构成、循行分布、生理机能、病理变化、脏腑形体官窍及精气血神，是指导人们疾病诊断与治疗的传统理论。

Ancient practitioners utilized methods such as acupuncture, guidance, massage, and Qigong for treatment and health maintenance. Based on anatomical knowledge at the time, they observed the phenomena of meridian sensation transmission in physiological and pathological states. Through repeated observations and summarizations in long-term medical practices, they developed the theory of meridians. This theory, developed under the guidance of Yin-Yang and Five Elements theories, is an essential component of traditional Chinese medicine. It encompasses the constitution, distribution, physiological functions, pathological changes, and the relationship between the viscera, meridians, and the essence, Qi, blood, and spirit of the human body. It serves as the traditional theoretical basis for guiding disease diagnosis and treatment.

According to the theory of the correspondence between the Five Elements and the internal organs and meridians, the six sounds "Xu", "He", "Hu", "Si", "Chui", and "Xi" respectively correspond to the liver, heart, spleen, lungs, kidneys, and triple energizer. Therefore, practicing the Liuzijue exercises has the effects of soothing the liver, regulating the spirit, invigorating the spleen, regulating the lungs, nourishing the kidneys, and regulating the triple energizer. By mastering the correct pronunciation, utilizing abdominal breathing, understanding key movements, grasping the principles of exertion, and following the seasonal sequences, one can enhance the effectiveness of strengthening the internal organs and toning the muscles and bones. The meridians and collaterals are distributed throughout the body, intricately connected, internally connected to the internal organs, externally linked to the joints, facilitating the circulation of Qi and blood, connecting the internal and external, and nourishing the organs and orifices. They integrate all the body's tissues and organs into an organic whole, transmit sensory information, coordinate Yin and Yang, and

根据五行与脏腑经络对应关系理论,"嘘""呵""呼""呬""吹""嘻"六个字分别与肝、心、脾、肺、肾、三焦相对应,故练习六字诀具有疏肝、调神、健脾、调肺、补肾、调理三焦的作用。掌握正确吐音,运用顺腹式呼吸,把握动作要点,领会发力要领,顺应四时节序,可以起到强脏腑、健筋骨的功效。经络遍布于全身,错综联络,内属于脏腑,外络于肢节,通行气血,沟通上下内外,濡养形体官窍,将机体所有的组织和器官联系成为有机的整体,感应、传导信息,协调阴阳,保证人体正常生命活动。

ensure the normal life activities of the human body.

第三节　气血学说
Section 3　The Theory of Qi and Blood

气者，人之根本也。《黄帝内经》说："人以天地之气，四时之法成。"说明气是构成和维持人体生命活动的基本物质，遵循四时气候更迭的运行规律，可以影响人体的生理、病理及疾病的预防。六字诀通过呼吸吐纳自然清气，按四时之季节练习来调动五脏和三焦之气，能更好地维持人体生命活动。人体气机畅通和协调平衡的状态，称为"气机调畅"，是人体生命活动正常的标志。气是运行不息的，是人体内不断升降出入运动的精微物质，是推动和调控脏腑生理机能的动力。《黄帝内经》也指出"顺应季节阴阳变化"。

Qi is the fundamental essence of a person. Huangdi's Classic on Medicine states: "Humans are formed by the Qi of heaven and earth, and follow the laws of the four seasons." This indicates that Qi is the fundamental substance that constitutes and maintains the life activities of the human body. Following the laws of the changing seasons and climate, Qi can influence the physiology, pathology, and prevention of diseases in the human body. The Liuzijue, through breathing regulation and natural Qi emission, practices according to the seasons to mobilize the Qi of the five internal organs and the triple energizer, thereby better maintaining the life activities of the human body. A state where the Qi flows smoothly and is balanced and coordinated is called "smooth circulation of Qi," which is a sign of normal life activities in the human body. Qi is constantly in motion, it is the subtle substance that continuously ascends, descends, and circulates within the body, and it is the driving force that propels and regulates the physiological functions of the organs. *Huangdi's Classic on Medicine* also points out the importance of adapting to the changes of Yin and Yang according to the seasons.

Qi and blood can stimulate and regulate the body's metabolism, driving the vital activities of the human body. In the practice of Liuzijue, by exercising the movement of one's own Qi through ascending, descending, entering, and exiting, one can enhance the ability to sustain vital activities.

气与血可以激发和调控机体的新陈代谢，推动人体生命活动。在六字诀的锻炼中，通过对自身之气的升降出入的运动锻炼，提高维持人体生命活动的能力。

第四节 人体运动学
Section 4 Human Kinesiology

Human kinetics is a discipline that studies the laws of motion of human activities or specific parts of the body, including their position, force, velocity, acceleration, etc. It involves various aspects such as the musculoskeletal system, respiratory system, and nervous system. It emphasizes the relationship between human movement and mechanics, physiology, and pathology. The bodily movements in Liuzijue conform to basic forms of human

人体运动学是研究人体活动或特定部位的位置、力、速度、加速度等运动规律的一门学科，涉及运动系统、呼吸系统和神经系统等多个方面，注重人体运动与力学、生理、病理之间的变化关系。六字诀的肢体动作符合摆动、躯干扭转、相向运动等人体的基本运动形式，以及通过六种不同的发音口型动作及唇齿喉舌的用力不同，可以改善体内之气的升降出入，从而影响人体的运动、力量、协调性和整体健康。

六字诀锻炼能改善人体肺的通气功能，提高呼吸耐力及最大摄氧量，加强呼吸功能，增强机体的运动能力，加快康复速度。虽然肺部的结构尚未观察到显著变化，但是对肺功能还是有显著改善作用。此功法动作具有动中有静、静中有动的特点，而且没有高强度锻炼带来的外伤和心脑血管风险。六字诀作为中国传统的健身气功之一，长期锻炼后对慢性阻塞性肺气肿（COPD）、支气管哮喘、慢性支气管炎、冠心病、便秘、肠易激综合征、功能性消化不良和骨质疏松症等常见疾病，均具有良好的防治效果，对于不同年龄段的人均有强身健体的作用。

movement such as swinging, trunk rotation, and reciprocal motion. Through six different pronunciations and variations in the force exerted by the lips, teeth, throat, and tongue, Liuzijue can improve the ascending, descending, entering, and exiting of Qi within the body, thereby affecting human movement, strength, coordination, and overall health.

The practice of Liuzijue can improve pulmonary ventilation function, enhance respiratory endurance and maximal oxygen uptake, strengthen respiratory function, enhance the body's physical capabilities, accelerate recovery speed. Although significant changes in lung structure have not been observed, there is a notable improvement in lung function. This practice involves both dynamic and static elements and does not carry the risk of external injuries or cardiovascular risks associated with high-intensity exercise. As one of the traditional Chinese health Qigong exercises, long-term practice of Liuzijue has shown positive effects in the prevention and treatment of common diseases such as chronic obstructive pulmonary disease (COPD), bronchial asthma, chronic bronchitis, coronary heart disease, constipation, irritable bowel syndrome, functional dyspepsia, and osteoporosis. It serves as an effective method for improving health and fitness for individuals of different age groups.

第三章 六字诀的特点

古代流传下来的六字诀中呼气吐字有六种变化,所以有六种字诀的姿势及锻炼方法,即嘘字诀、呵字诀、呼字诀、呬字诀、吹字诀、嘻字诀。本书采用的六字诀招式名称与之相同。

Chapter 3 Characteristics of Liuzijue

In the ancient tradition of Liuzijue, there are six variations of exhaling and vocalizing, resulting in six different postures and exercise methods. These are known as the "Xu" posture, "He" posture, "Hu" posture, "Si" posture, "Chui" posture, and "Xi" posture. These names correspond to the techniques used in this book for practicing Liuzijue.

第一节 平衡阴阳
Section 1　Balancing Yin and Yang

六字诀是中国传统气功修炼方法之一，在中医阴阳五行、生克制化等中医基础理论的指导下，通过呼吸、发声和动作锻炼，调节五脏和三焦的阴阳，以达到人体阴阳的动态平衡。在呼吸锻炼方面，呼气的时候是阳，吸气的时候是阴，阳亢体质者多呼以潜阳，阴虚体质者多吸以滋阴。在六字诀动作导引上，向上、向外的为阳，可以提升阳气；向下、向里的为阴，可以滋阴潜阳。六字诀功法对外锻炼躯体、四肢的肌肉力量及协调性，具有调形作用；对内锻炼呼吸肌及辅助肌群，如膈肌、肋间肌、腹肌、斜角肌及胸锁乳突肌等参加呼吸运动，具有调气作用；内外兼修，提高身体的呼吸功能、运动功能，体现以形引气、以气导形的功效。

Liuzijue is one of the traditional Qigong practices in China. Guided by the fundamental theories of Traditional Chinese Medicine, such as the theory of Yin and Yang and the Five Elements, it aims to regulate the Yin and Yang of the five viscera and triple energizer through breathing, vocalization, and movements, thereby achieving dynamic balance in the human body's Yin and Yang. In terms of respiratory exercise, exhaling represents Yang, while inhaling represents Yin. Those with excessive Yang constitution tend to focus on exhaling to subdue Yang, while those with Yin deficiency tend to focus on inhaling to nourish Yin. Regarding the guiding principle of the movements in Liuzijue, upward and outward movements represent Yang, which can elevate Yang Qi; downward and inward movements represent Yin, which can nourish Yin and subdue Yang. The practice of Liuzijue exercises the muscles and coordination of the body's trunk and limbs externally, thereby influencing body shape. Internally, it exercises the respiratory muscles and auxiliary muscle groups, such as the diaphragm, intercostal muscles, abdominal muscles, oblique muscles, and pectoralis minor, which participate in breathing movements, thereby regulating Qi. By simultaneously focusing on internal and external aspects, it enhances the body's respiratory and motor functions, reflecting the effectiveness of guiding Qi through form and form through Qi.

In clinical practice, we often encounter patients' symptoms such as headaches, dizziness, insomnia, neck pain, back pain, waist pain, chest tightness, anxiety, nervousness, emotional tension, and functional digestive disorders, often caused by work, study, and psychological stress. These symptoms are mainly caused by prolonged periods of poor posture, such as sitting with the head down, and a lack of rest and exercise, leading to weakening of the core muscle groups in the chest, abdomen, and back, as well as affecting the function of the respiratory muscles. When abnormal body postures such as rounded shoulders and hunched backs occur, they further affect the patient's mental state, leading to anxiety, depression, and feelings of inferiority. During the practice of Liuzijue, each vocalized sound corresponds to a specific organ and guides the breath to that organ, helping to release accumulated stress or energy, regulate the body's breath, promote blood circulation, and adjust the Yin and Yang of the internal organs. "Xu"

临床上，经常碰到因工作、学习和心理压力，导致的头痛、头晕、失眠、颈痛、背痛、腰痛、胸闷、焦虑不安、情绪紧张、功能性消化不良等不适症状。基本上都是由于长时间保持久坐低头的不良姿势习惯，缺乏休息和运动，以至于胸腹部及腰背部的核心肌群减弱，也影响到呼吸肌群的功能。当出现圆肩驼背、高低肩等异常体态后，会进一步影响患者的心理，产生焦虑不安、情绪抑郁及自卑感等情志病。在锻炼六字诀的过程中，每个吐字都有独特的发声，将气息引导至相应的内脏器官，以帮助释放积聚的压力或能量，调节体内的气息，促进血液循环，调节内脏器官的阴阳。

"嘘"属肝木，可以去肝脏积热、泻肝脏浊气、减少愤怒、减轻压力，改善肝脏功能；"呵"属心火，可以去心火、缓解焦虑紧张，改善心功能；"呼"属脾土，泻脾胃浊气、增强消化功能；"呬"属肺金，泻肺脏浊气、改善肺功能；"吹"属肾水，泻肾脏浊气、减少多余的水分，改善肾功能；"嘻"声通过三焦，畅通全身气血，调节气息与平衡阴阳。长期锻炼六字诀可以增强身体肌肉力量及平衡性、减少压力、提高注意力、增强免疫、缓解焦虑紧张和促进情绪的稳定，并在整体上促进身体和精神的和谐。

corresponds to the Liver Wood, which can clear Liver heat, disperse Liver stagnation, reduce anger, alleviate stress to improve Liver function; "He" corresponds to the Heart Fire, which can clear Heart Fire, relieve anxiety and tension to improve Heart function; "Hu" corresponds to the Spleen Earth, which can disperse Spleen and Stomach turbidity to enhance digestive function; "Si" corresponds to the Lung Metal, which can disperse Lung turbidity to improve Lung function; "Chui" corresponds to the Kidney Water, which can disperse Kidney turbidity, reduce excess water to improve Kidney function; "Xi" sound through the triple energizer, promotes the smooth flow of Qi and blood throughout the body, regulates breath, and balances Yin and Yang. Long-term practice of Liuzijue has been found to enhance muscle strength and balance, reduce stress, improve attention, strengthen immunity, alleviate anxiety and tension, promote emotional stability, and overall, promote harmony between body and mind.

第二节 内敛精神
Section 2　Cultivating Inner Spirit

Liuzijue's breathing and movement guidance method is used to adjust and control the ascending, descending, entering, and exiting of internal Qi, regulate internal intention and Qi, balance the Yin and Yang of the organs, and achieve the unity of mental adjustment and physical strengthening. Liuzijue emphasizes the importance of "intentional cultivation of Qi, with Qi following intention, and intention and Qi mutually following each other." It values the significant role of "intention." "Intention" refers to the rhythmic regulation of autonomous activity that occurs after the cerebral cortex enters a deep-state of function activation, representing a mild state of active mental activity and the potential activation of deep brain functions. Liuzijue exercises involve using one's own intentions to influence the internal movements of breath and Qi, aligning the movements of breath and Qi within the body with mental activities. This helps the practitioner to concentrate, maintain a tranquil mind, eliminate distractions, experience the coordination and naturalness of bodily movements, breathing, and vocalization,

六字诀功法的呼吸吐纳，配合动作导引，可以调整和控制体内气息的升降出入，调节内在意和气，平衡脏腑阴阳，达到调神和强身的统一。六字诀讲究"意守炼气，气随意行，意气相随"，重视"意念"的重要地位。"意念"是人体大脑皮层入静后深层功能激发产生的自主能动的节律性调控，潜在脑功能的轻度活跃精神状态。六字诀锻炼是用自己的意念活动来影响内在的呼吸和气息的运动，使体内的气息运动和意念活动一致；使锻炼者注意力集中，思想安宁，排除杂念，体会到肢体动作、呼吸、吐音协调自然，锻炼大脑对中枢神经和外周本体感觉，加强对身体和精神的自我控制。

六字诀的吐气发音训练，首先要掌握正确的吐音，刚开始训练时应该发出声音以自己耳朵听到的声量为度，熟练后的声量可以逐渐减小到不发出声音，以发出气息为主，感知身体内脏与声音共振即可。早期的"意念"训练是刻意的，有意为之的，需要有意识的思维训练，不断地提醒自己激发潜意识，通过不断地学习和训练，"意念"将成为人体大脑对自己身体和外界的自然反应，无限接近本能反应，而不需要刻意思考。由意念引导呼吸之气，有意识地调节呼吸，将呼吸、发声与动作姿势结合起来，通过反复训练，由意识强化逐渐过渡到自然松弛状态。如锻炼"呬"字诀时，口吐"呬"字音，同时松肩伸项，两掌向前平推，先意想如缓缓推开窗户，意有排山之势。两掌外旋，屈肘，同时两掌缓缓收拢至胸前，意想潮水缓缓退

and exercise the brain's central nervous system and peripheral proprioception, thereby strengthening self-control over the body and mind.

The exhalation vocalization training of Liuzijue begins with mastering the correct vocalization. At the initial stages of training, the sound should be produced at a volume that is audible to oneself. With proficiency, the volume can gradually decrease until no sound is emitted, focusing mainly on the exhalation of breath. It's important to perceive the resonance between the internal organs and the sound. Early "intention" training is deliberate and conscious, requiring deliberate thought and conscious mental training. Continuously reminding oneself to stimulate the subconscious mind is necessary. After continuous learning and training, "intention" will become a natural response of the human brain to one's own body and the external environment, approaching an instinctive response without the need for deliberate thought. Guided by intention, the breath is consciously regulated, combining breathing, vocalization, and movement postures. Through repeated training, one gradually transitions from conscious reinforcement to a state of natural relaxation. For example, in practicing the "Si" posture, one vocalizes the "Si" sound while relaxing the shoulders, extending the neck, and pushing both palms forward slowly, imagining the gradual opening of a window with force. Then, both palms rotate outward, elbows bend, while simultaneously and slowly retracting both palms towards the chest, imagining the gradual receding of the tide. Through such repetitive training and guided meditation through breath control and vocalization, the integration of body movements and intentions becomes natural and coordinated, helping to internalize the spirit, reduce external interference, and achieve a state of "movement following intention, intention following one's desire".

第三节 调整呼吸
Section 3　Adjusting Breathing

The breathing exercise method of Liuzijue integrates pursed-lip breathing, abdominal breathing, and bodily movements, primarily training breathing and vocal sounds. Exhaling while uttering the sounds six of "Xu, He, Hu, Si, Chui, and Xi" involves various mouth shapes and different exertions of the lips teech, throat and tongue, each of which affects the five viscera and the triple energizer respectively.

Liuzijue employs abdominal breathing,

吸，可改变异常呼吸模式，提高潮气量，先呼后吸，呼吸要求做到"匀、细、柔、长"。呼气时，腹部收缩，吐字发声均匀柔长，同时提肛、收小腹、缩臀；吸气时经鼻，腹部膨胀，每次吸气后不要忙于呼出，宜稍屏片刻，再徐徐呼出。这种呼吸方式可以加大膈肌的收缩与舒张，增强横膈膜的力量，增加肺部容量，提高呼吸器官血液循环，促进氧气吸收，从而改善肺功能。再通过不同的发音在人体腹腔内产生不同的内压，循经导引，引导人体气血沿着各脏腑对应的经络运行，调节全身各脏腑功能，从而达到提高肺的免疫功能及增强肺功能的目的。

现代医学认为，呼吸训练对呼气肌和吸气肌有

which can alter abnormal breathing patterns, increase tidal volume, and emphasizes exhalation before inhalation. The breathing requirements include being "even, fine, gentle, and long". When one exhales, the abdomen contracts, and vocalization of the sounds is even, gentle, and prolonged. Simultaneously, the anus is tightened, the lower abdomen is pulled in, and the buttocks are contracted. Inhale through the nose, and the abdomen expands. After each inhalation, one should not rush to exhale but rather hold the breath for a moment before slowly exhaling. This breathing technique can enhance the contraction and relaxation of the diaphragm, strengthen the diaphragmatic muscles, increase lung capacity, improve the circulation of blood in respiratory organs, facilitate oxygen absorption, and thereby improve lung function. Furthermore, through the production of different internal pressures in the abdominal cavity via different vocalizations, and through channeling along the corresponding meridians, the circulation of Qi and blood is guided along the meridians corresponding to various visceral organs, regulating the functions of the whole body's visceral organs. This ultimately aims to enhance the immune function of the lungs and strengthen lung function.

Modern medicine believes that respiratory training imposes a certain resistance load on the expiratory and inspiratory muscles, resulting in an increase in breathing rate, depth, and lung ventilation during the exercise. This not only enhances the strength and endurance of respiratory muscles but also improves the mobility of the chest wall, providing exercise and strengthening for the respiratory organs. Pursed-lip breathing can shift the equal pressure point towards the central airway, preventing premature closure of small airways, making it easier to expel residual air from the lungs, increasing alveolar ventilation, reducing respiratory workload, improving oxygen tolerance, and alleviating symptoms of respiratory difficulty.

一定阻力负荷，使运动时呼吸数增加、深度加深、肺通气量增加，不仅可以增强呼吸肌肌力和耐力，也可增强胸廓活动性，呼吸器官得到锻炼和增强。缩唇呼吸，可使等压点移向中央气道，防止小气道过早闭合，使肺内残气更易于排出，增加肺泡通气量，降低呼吸功耗，提高耐氧能力，缓解呼吸困难症状。

第四节　变易筋骨
Section 4　Transforming Muscles and Bones

The function of Liuzijue in transforming and strengthening muscles and bones focuses on adjusting breathing and body movements to promote the flexibility, agility, and strength of tendons and bones. By combining vocalization, breathing, and movement, it influences the body's musculoskeletal structure. Deep breathing and abdominal breathing can help

六字诀变易筋骨的作用集中于通过调整呼吸和身体动作，来促进筋骨的柔韧性、灵活性和力量。通过发声、呼吸和动作的结合，来影响身体的筋骨结构。深呼吸和腹式呼吸可以帮助锻炼者放松肌肉，减少关节的僵硬，促进关节的灵活性。深呼吸还可以增加氧气的吸收，促进血液循环，这对增强筋骨的力量和灵活性至关重要。每个音节的发声都需要练习者使用特定的肌肉和呼吸方式，这有助于增强肌肉的力量，如膈肌、胸锁乳突肌及胸腹部肌群等，改善肺通气功能，提高呼吸耐力，加强呼吸功能，从而改善肺循环。

身体动作在六字诀中也非常重要，它们可以帮助练习者调整身体的姿态，增强身体运动能量，促进身体的平衡，可以降低受伤的风险。比如，"嘘"声对应肝脏，肝在体合筋，肝脏与筋骨的柔韧性有关；"呼"声对应脾脏，脾在体合肉，脾脏与肌肉的力量相关。通过练习这些音节，练习者可以增强相应器官的功能，进而促进筋骨的健康。

除了对身体运动能力、承受能力及协调性的影响，六字诀还可以通过调整呼吸和发声来促进心理和精

practitioners relax muscles, reduce joint stiffness, and promote joint flexibility. Deep breathing also enhances oxygen absorption and promotes blood circulation, which is crucial for strengthening the strength and flexibility of tendons and bones. Each syllable requires practitioners to use specific muscles and breathing techniques, which helps strengthen muscles such as the diaphragm, pectoralis major, and chest and abdominal muscles, improving lung ventilation function, enhancing respiratory endurance, strengthening respiratory function, and thus improving lung circulation.

Body movements are also crucial in Liuzijue, as they help practitioners adjust their posture, enhance physical energy, promote balance, and reduce the risk of injury. For example, the "Xu" sound corresponds to the Liver, which governs tendons in the body, and is related to the flexibility of tendons and bones; the "Hu" sound corresponds to the Spleen, which governs muscles in the body, and is related to muscle strength. By practicing these syllables, practitioners can strengthen the functions of corresponding organs, thereby promoting the health of tendons and bones.

In addition to its impact on physical abilities, endurance, and coordination, Liuzijue can also promote mental and spiritual health through adjusting breathing and vocalization. By regulating breathing, practitioners can achieve a calm and relaxed state, which is crucial for mental well-being. Specific vocalizations can help practitioners focus their attention and enhance mental resilience.

神的健康。通过调整呼吸，练习者可以达到平静和放松的状态，这对心理健康非常重要。特定的发声可以帮助练习者集中注意力，增强心理韧性。

第四章 ● 六字诀分步解析

六字诀呼吸吐纳功法套路锻炼中需要牢记习练要点：精神内守、思想集中，与吐音、呼吸、动作配合协调自然；动作要尽量放松，自然站立，两肘、膝关节微屈；顺腹式呼吸、先呼后吸，呼气时读字，同时提肛、收小腹、缩臀，重心后移至脚跟，脚趾轻微点地；吸气时嘴唇轻闭，舌抵上颚，空气自然吸入，腹部自然隆起，达到松、静、自然。

Chapter 4　Step-by-Step Analysis of Liuzijue

In practicing the breathing and vocalization techniques of Liuzijue, it's important to bear key points in mind: mental focus and concentration, coordination with breathing, vocalization, and movements in a natural and harmonious manner. All movements should be as relaxed as possible, maintaining a natural standing posture, with slightly bent elbows and knee joints. Practice abdominal breathing, exhaling before inhaling, vocalizing during exhalation, while simultaneously contracting the anus, pulling in the lower abdomen, and tightening the buttocks. Shift the body weight to the heels, with the toes lightly touching the ground. when inhaling, lightly close the lips, place the tongue against the palate, allowing air to naturally enter, with the abdomen naturally rising, achieving a state of relaxation, stillness, and naturalness.

预 备 式
Preparatory Posture

【动作描述】

自然站立,两脚分开,与肩同宽,身体正直,虚领顶劲,嘴唇轻闭,舌抵上颚,下颌微收,含胸拔背,松腰收腹,两臂自然下垂,中指贴于裤缝,两膝微曲,心平气和,面带微笑,全身放松(图1、图2)。

[Description of the Movement]

Stand naturally with feet shoulder-width apart, maintaining an upright posture, and keeping the body aligned. Lift the crown of the head slightly as if suspended from above, lightly close the lips, place the tongue against the palate, slightly retract the lower jaw, tuck in the chin, lift the chest, and straighten the back. Relax the waist and pull in the abdomen gently. Let the arms hang naturally by the sides, with the middle fingers lightly touching the seam of the

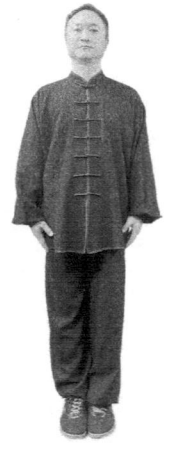

图 1
Fig.1

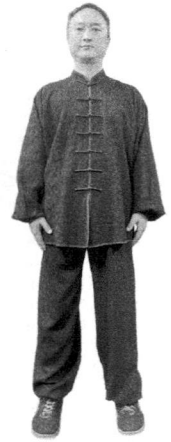

图 2
Fig.2

pants. Keep the knees slightly bent, maintain a calm and gentle demeanor, wear a slight smile on the face, and ensure the entire body is relaxed (Fig. 1, Fig. 2).

第一式 "嘘" 字诀
One "Xu" Zijue

扫码看视频

[Pronunciation and Mouth Shape]

The sound "Xu" for the character "Xū" (pronounced as " 需 ," with a flat tone), belongs to the dental consonants. When exhaling and producing sound, slightly open the lips and teeth, purse the lips, and gently exhale the air from the gaps between the molars and the sides of the tongue, releasing it slowly outward.

[Description of the Movement]

The body turns 90° to the left while the right palm is extended to the left side of the body at shoulder height, with the mouth pronouncing the sound "Xu". The eyes are wide open, focusing on the right palm. The right palm then slowly returns to the waist as the body returns to the forward position, with the gaze directed downward in front. Repeat the same movements on the opposite side. Alternate between the left and right sides, practicing six times in total.

【发音与口型】

"嘘"字音"xū"（读需，音平），属牙音。发声吐气时，两唇和牙齿微张开，缩唇，气从槽牙间、舌两边的空隙缓缓呼出体外。

【动作描述】

身体向左侧转动 90°，同时右掌朝上向身体左侧伸出，与肩平齐，并配合口吐"嘘"字音，眼睛睁大，双眼注视右掌；右掌缓缓收回腰间，同时身体回正，目视前下方。左右交换，动作要领相同，方向相反。如此左右交替练习六遍。

【分步练习】

（1）预备式（图3）。

（2）重心在右脚，左脚向左侧开一步，两手松开，掌心朝上，双手小指轻贴于腰间，两脚不动。身体向左转动90°，同时右掌缓缓向身体左侧伸出，与肩平齐，并配合口吐"嘘"字音，眼睛随之慢慢睁大，双眼注视右掌伸出方向。

（3）右掌沿原路慢慢收回腰间，同时身体随之转回正前方，目视前下方（图4）。

（4）然后，身体向右转动90°，左掌从腰间缓缓向身体右侧伸出，与肩平齐，并配合口吐"嘘"字音，动作及要领与前相同，但方向相反，全身松静自然。如此左右交替反复练习六遍（图5）。

（5）最后，两肩放松，两上肢自然落下垂于体侧，中指贴于裤缝，左脚收回，目视前下方，静养片刻，恢复预备式。

[Step-by-Step Practice]

(1) Preparation posture (Fig. 3).

(2) Shift your weight onto your right foot, and step to the left with your left foot. Relax your hands, turning your palms upward, and lightly place the little fingers against your waist. Without moving your feet, turn your body 90° to the left while slowly extending your right palm to the left side of your body at shoulder height. Simultaneously, exhale the sound "Xu," and gradually widen your eyes, focusing on the direction your right palm is extending.

(3) Slowly retract your right palm along the same path back to your waist while turning your body back to the forward position, with your gaze directed downward in front (Fig. 4).

(4) Next, turn your body 90° to the right. Extend your left palm slowly from your waist to the right side of your body at shoulder height while exhaling the sound "Xu." The movements and key points are the same as before, but in the opposite direction. Keep your whole body relaxed and natural. Repeat this alternating practice six times on each side (Fig. 5).

(5) Finally, relax both shoulders and let your arms naturally fall to your sides, with your middle fingers touching the seams of your pants. Bring your left foot back in, gaze downward in front, rest quietly for a moment, and return to the preparation

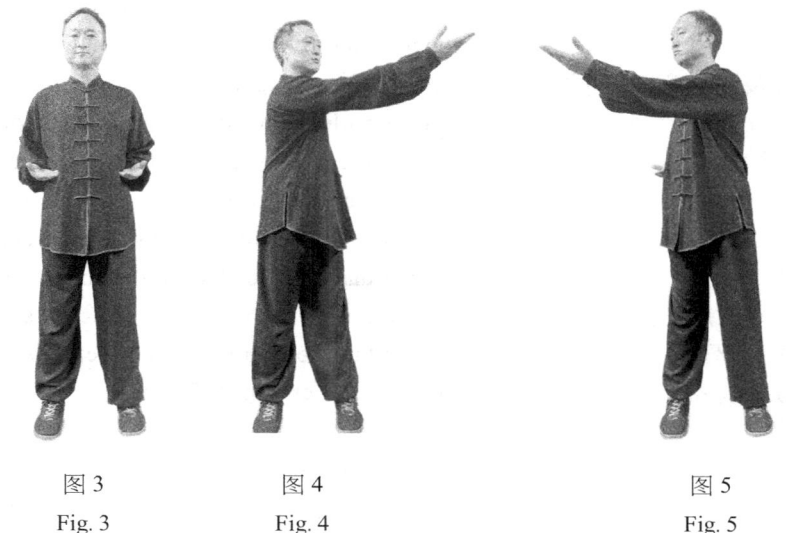

| 图 3 | 图 4 | 图 5 |
| Fig. 3 | Fig. 4 | Fig. 5 |

posture.

[Musculoskeletal Characteristics]

(1) Pay attention to the exhalation and mouth shape while producing the "Xu" sound, not excessively emphasizing mental focus, maintaining a natural and coordinated approach.

(2) Rotate the body approximately 90° to the left or right without lifting the feet off the ground.

(3) As one palm slowly extends to the side, let your eyes follow the direction of the extending palm, keeping the elbow joints relaxed, and focused attention.

[Health Cultivation Elements]

The "Xu" sound corresponds to the liver among the five internal organs. Spring

【肌骨特征】

（1）注意"嘘"字音的发声吐气及口型，不必过分强调意念，保持自然协调。

（2）身体左右转动约90°，两脚不动，不可离地。

（3）当一掌向一侧徐徐伸出时，双眼要跟随掌伸出的方向，肘关节放松，注意力要集中。

【养生要素】

"嘘"字功与五脏之肝脏相对应，春嘘明目木扶肝，春季多练，具有疏通气机、清肝明目、濡养肝及筋目和调理肝脏功能的作用。此功法动作着重锻炼胁肋、腰背、四肢经筋。

可用于肝火旺、肝阴虚、眩晕、中风昏厥、眼疾，或情志抑郁、焦虑，或两胁肋部疼痛、胃脘痞闷、嗳气泛恶、腹痛腹泻等疾病的防治和康复。也可作颈椎病、肩周炎、腰背部筋膜炎等病症的传统导引方法。

is associated with the "Xu" exercise, which supports the liver's function of nourishing the eyes. Practicing during the spring season can help clear the liver, improve vision, nourish the liver and tendons, and regulate liver function. This exercise primarily focuses on exercising the ribs, waist, back, the meridians and tendons of the limbs.

It can be used to prevent and rehabilitate conditions such as excessive liver fire, liver Yin deficiency, dizziness, stroke-induced fainting, eye disorders, as well as emotional issues like depression and anxiety. Additionally, it can help alleviate ailments like rib pain, gastric discomfort, belching, abdominal pain, and diarrhea. Furthermore, it serves as a traditional guiding method for conditions such as cervical spondylosis, shoulder periarthritis, and fasciitis in the lumbar region.

第二式 "呵"字诀
Two "He" Zijue

扫码看视频

【发音与口型】

"呵"字音"hē"（读喝，音平），属舌音。发声吐气时，两唇和牙齿微张开，缩唇，气从舌与上

[Pronunciation and Mouth Shape]

The sound "He" for the character "hē", (pronounced like "喝" with a flat tone), belongs to tongue consonants. When exhaling and producing the sound, gently part the lips and teeth, with the lips slightly puckered. Exhale gently through the gap between the tongue and the palate of the mouth.

[Description of the Movement]

With both palms slightly raised and fingertips pointing diagonally downwards, squat down while bending the knees. Simultaneously, extend both palms forward and downward at about a 45° angle, bending the elbows and retracting the arms. The palms should be close together with the little fingers touching, and the palms facing upward as if holding something. Position the palms in front of the abdomen, gaze at the center of the palms, and gradually straighten both knees while bending the elbows. Bring both palms towards the chest, rotating them so that the palms face inward, with the middle fingers roughly level with the lower jaw, and the elbows slightly outward and level with the shoulders. Rotate the palms inward so that the fingertips point downward and the backs of the hands are close together. Slowly lower the palms while exhaling the sound "He". When the palms are level with the navel, slightly bend the knees again, rotate the palms inward with the palms facing outward, and gently push both arms forward, forming a circular motion. For the second repetition, rotate the palms outward as if holding something, and then repeat the previous movements. Do

腭之间缓缓呼出体外。

【动作描述】

两掌微微上提，指尖朝向斜下方，屈膝下蹲，同时两掌缓缓向前下约45°方向插出；屈肘收臂，两掌小指相靠，掌心向上呈捧掌，于腹部前，目视两掌心，两膝缓缓伸直；同时屈肘，两掌捧至胸前，转成掌心向内，两中指约与下颌等高，两肘外展，与肩同高；两掌内翻，掌指朝下，掌背相靠，缓缓下插，同时口吐"呵"字音。两掌下插至与肚脐相平时，微屈膝下蹲，两掌内旋，掌心向外，缓缓向前拨出两臂成圆。第二遍两掌外旋呈捧掌，然后重复前面的动作，如此重复练习六遍。

【分步练习】
（1）接上式。

（2）两掌微微上提，掌心朝上，五指并拢，指尖朝向斜下方，屈膝下蹲，同时两掌缓缓向前下约45°插出，双侧肘、膝关节放松（图6）。

（3）屈肘收臂，两掌靠拢，两掌小指侧相靠，掌心向上呈捧掌，约与脐平，目视两掌心，两膝缓缓伸直，同时屈肘，两掌捧至胸前，与乳平，转成掌心向内，两中指约与下颌同高，两肘外展，与肩同高，两掌内翻，掌指朝下，掌背相靠，缓缓下插，同时口吐"呵"字音（图7）。

（4）两掌下插至与脐平时，微屈膝下蹲，两掌内旋，掌心向外，缓缓向前拨出两臂成圆。第二遍两掌向外旋转呈捧掌，然后重复前面的动作，如此

this exercise six times.

[Step-by-Step Practice]

(1) Continue from the previous exercise.

(2) With both palms slightly raised, palms facing upward, fingers together, and fingertips pointing diagonally downwards, squat down while bending the knees. Simultaneously, extend both palms forward and downward at about a 45° angle, keeping the elbows and knees relaxed (Fig. 6).

(3) Bend the elbows and retract the arms, bringing the palms close together with the little fingers touching. The palms should be facing upward as if holding something, roughly level with the navel. Gaze at the center of the palms, gradually straighten both knees while bending the elbows. Bring both palms towards the chest, with the palms facing inward, and the middle fingers roughly level with the lower jaw. Keep the elbows slightly outward and level with the shoulders. Rotate the palms inward so that the fingertips point downward, and the backs of the hands are close together. Slowly lower the palms while exhaling the sound "He" (Fig. 7).

(4) When the palms are level with the navel, slightly bend the knees again, rotate the palms inward with the palms facing outward, and gently push both arms forward, forming a circular motion. For the second repetition, rotate the palms outward

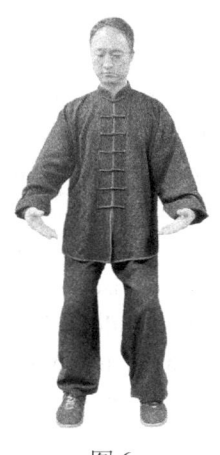 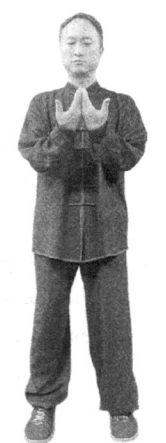 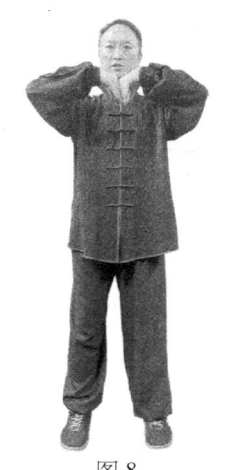

图 6　　　　　图 7　　　　　图 8
Fig. 6　　　　Fig. 7　　　　Fig. 8

as if holding something, and then repeat the previous movements. Do this exercise six times. (Fig. 8)

[Musculoskeletal Characteristics]

(1) Ensure that the knees do not extend beyond the toes, and maintain stability in the center of gravity.

(2) Coordinate the gradual straightening of both knees with the lifting of both palms, ensuring a natural movement.

(3) As the palms point downward and lower slowly, try to keep the elbow joints as straight as possible, extending outward and stretching, level with the shoulders, without hunching the back or rounding the shoulders.

[Health Cultivation Elements]

The exercise associated with the "He" sound corresponds to the Heart among the

重复练习六遍（图 8）。

【肌骨特征】

（1）屈膝下蹲时，膝关节不能超出足尖，重心要稳。

（2）两膝缓缓伸直的同时，与两掌上抬协调自然。

（3）两掌指朝下，缓缓下插时，两肘关节尽量伸直、外展拉伸，与肩同高，不能含胸驼背。

【养生要素】

"呵"字功与五脏之心脏相应，心与夏季相通应。夏季多练,具有疏通心经、调神志、调血脉和调理心脏功能的作用。此功法动作着重锻炼肩关节、腕关节、四肢经筋。

可用于心悸、高血压、心阳虚衰、情志病、失眠、健忘、舌体糜烂等疾病的防治和康复。也可作为肩关节周围炎、腕关节疼痛、膝骨关节炎等病症的传统导引方法。

five internal organs, and the heart corresponds to the summer season. Exercising more during the summer helps regulate the heart fire naturally. Practicing during the summer season is beneficial for clearing the heart meridian, regulating emotions, balancing blood circulation, and nurturing heart health. This exercise method focuses on exercising the shoulder joints, wrist joints, and the meridians of the limbs.

It can be utilized for prevention and rehabilitation of conditions such as palpitations, hypertension, deficiency of heart Yang, emotional disorders, insomnia, forgetfulness, and lingual ulceration. Additionally, it can serve as a traditional guiding method for conditions like periarthritis of the shoulder, wrist joint pain, and knee osteoarthritis.

第三式 "呼"字诀
Three "Hu" Zijue

扫码看视频

【发音与口型】

"呼"字音"hū"(读乎,音平),属喉音。发声吐气时,口唇撮圆,舌体稍下沉,气从喉出后,在口腔形成一股中间气流,

[Pronunciation and Mouth Shape]

The sound "Hu" (pronounced " 乎 ", flat tone) is a guttural sound. When one makes the sound and exhaling, the lips should be rounded, the tongue slightly lowered, and the breath should come from the throat, forming a central airflow in the mouth, which is then expelled through the rounded lips.

[Description of the Movement]

Continuing from the previous posture, after both palms are extended forward, rotate them outward, and slowly bring the palms together in front of the navel. As you squat down and bend your knees, exhale with the sound "Hu", while both palms push outward, forming a ball-holding posture in front of the navel. Then bring the palms together again, push outward, and repeat this practice six times.

[Step-by-Step Practice]

(1) Continuing from the previous posture.

(2) After both palms are extended forward, rotate them outward, with the palms facing inward towards the abdomen. As you slowly straighten your knees, move the palms together slowly to a point about 10 cm in front of the navel (Fig. 9).

(3) As you slowly squat down and relax your hips and knees, exhale with the sound "Hu". At the same time, push both palms outward with palms facing inward, fingers naturally spread, forming a ball-holding posture in front of the navel. Look slightly downward in front of you, focusing your mind and regulating your breath (Fig. 10).

(4) Then, bring the palms together again, push outward, and repeat this practice

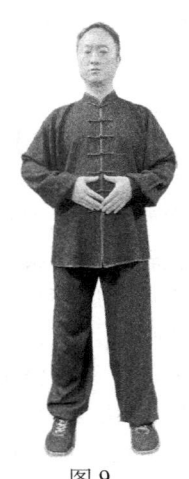

图 9
Fig. 9

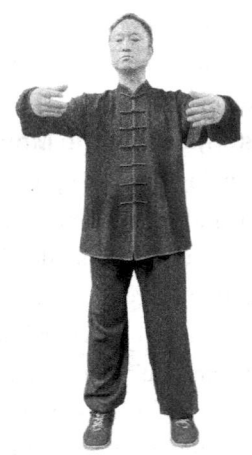

图 10
Fig. 10

【肌骨特征】

（1）两膝伸直与两掌合拢同时进行，重心要稳，呼吸自然。

（2）当两掌向外撑，掌心朝内，形成抱球姿势时，髋膝关节要自然放松，两手掌相距约15厘米，肘关节形成的夹角约120°。

（3）口吐"呼"字音时，微屈膝下蹲时，膝关节不能超出足尖。

【养生要素】

"呼"字功，与五脏之脾脏相对应，脾主四时，

six times.

[Musculoskeletal Characteristics]

(1) Straighten your knees while bringing your palms together simultaneously. Maintain balance and keep your breathing natural.

(2) When you push your palms outward with palms facing inward to form a ball-holding posture, naturally relax your hip and knee joints. Keep your palms about 15 cm apart, with the angle at your elbow joints around 120°.

(3) As you exhale with the sound "Hu" and slightly squat down, ensure that your knees do not go beyond your toes.

[Health Cultivation Elements]

The "Hu" sound corresponds to the Spleen among the five internal organs. The spleen governs all seasons, and prolonged exhalation benefits the spleen's digestive functions throughout the year. This exercise can be practiced in all seasons and is beneficial for strengthening the spleen, aiding digestion, clearing the spleen meridian, and regulating spleen function. The movements of this exercise focus on training the meridians and tendons of the shoulders, upper arms, wrists, and fingers.

It can be utilized for the prevention and rehabilitation of conditions such as spleen deficiency, abdominal distension, diarrhea, indigestion, and loss of appetite. Additionally, it can serve as a traditional guiding method for conditions such as periarthritis of the shoulder, chronic respiratory diseases, sarcopenia in the elderly, and weakness of the limbs.

四季长呼脾化餐。四季皆可练，具有健脾消食、疏通脾经、调理脾脏功能的作用。此功法动作着重锻炼肩部、上臂部、手腕部、掌指部的经筋。

可用于脾虚、腹胀、腹泻、消化不良、食欲不振等疾病的防治和康复。也可作为肩关节周围炎、慢性呼吸系统疾病、老年肌肉减少症、四肢乏力等病症的传统导引方法。

第四式 "呬"字诀
Four "Si" Zijue

[Pronunciation and Mouth Shape]

The sound "Si" (pronounced "四", flat tone) is a dental sound. When making the sound and exhaling, align the upper and lower front teeth, leaving a narrow gap. Lightly press the tip of the tongue against

【发音与口型】

"呬"字音"sī"（读四，音平），属齿音。发声吐气时，上下门牙对齐，留有狭缝，舌尖轻抵下齿，气从门牙齿间呼出体外。

【动作描述】

接上式，两膝缓缓伸直，同时，两掌自然下落，两掌缓缓向上托至胸前与乳平；两肘下落，夹肋，两手顺势立掌于肩前，掌心相对，指尖向上，两肩胛骨向脊柱靠拢，展肩扩胸，藏头缩项，目视前上方；微屈膝下蹲，口吐"呬"字音，同时松肩伸项，两掌缓缓向前平推，逐渐转成掌心向前亮掌，目视前方；两掌向外旋转，转成掌心向内，两膝缓缓伸直，同时屈肘，两掌缓缓收拢至胸前；然后再落肘，夹肋，立掌，展肩扩胸，藏头缩项，推掌，口吐"呬"字音，如此重复练习六遍。

【分步练习】

（1）接上式。

（2）两膝缓缓伸直，

the lower teeth, and expel the breath through the gap between the front teeth.

[Description of the Movement]

Continuing from the previous posture, slowly straighten your knees while letting your palms naturally fall, then slowly raise your palms up to chest level, aligning with your nipples. As your elbows drop and tuck in by your ribs, position your hands with palms facing each other and fingers pointing upward in front of your shoulders. Pull your shoulder blades toward the spine, expand your chest, tuck your head in, and look slightly upward. Slightly bend your knees and squat down, exhaling with the sound "Si". At the same time, relax your shoulders and extend your neck. Slowly push your palms forward, gradually turning them so that the palms face forward. Keep your eyes looking straight ahead. Rotate your palms outward so that they face inward again. As you slowly straighten your knees, bend your elbows, and gradually bring your palms back to your chest. Then, lower your elbows, tuck them by your ribs, position your hands with palms facing each other, expand your chest, tuck your head in, and push your palms forward, exhaling with the sound "Si". Repeat this practice six times.

[Step-by-Step Practice]

(1) Continuing from the previous posture.

(2) Slowly straighten your knees while

letting your palms naturally fall with palms facing upward and fingers pointing towards each other. Slowly raise your palms up to chest level, aligning with your nipples (Fig. 11).

(3) Drop your elbows and tuck them by your ribs, positioning your hands in front of your shoulders, with palms facing each other and fingers pointing upward. Pull your shoulder blades firmly towards the spine, expand your chest, tuck your head in without shrugging your shoulders, and look slightly upward with your eyes wide open (Fig. 12).

(4) Rotate your wrists outward so that the palms face inward. Slowly straighten your knees while bending your elbows, and gradually bring your palms back to your chest.

同时，两掌自然下落，掌心向上，十指相对，两掌缓缓向上托至胸前与乳平（图 11）。

（3）两肘下落，夹肋，两手顺势立掌于肩前，掌心相对，指尖向上，两肩胛骨用力向脊柱靠拢，展肩扩胸，藏头缩项，不要耸肩，目视前上方，眼睛睁大（图 12）。

（4）两掌外旋腕，转成掌心向内，两膝缓缓伸直，同时屈肘，两掌缓缓收拢至胸前。

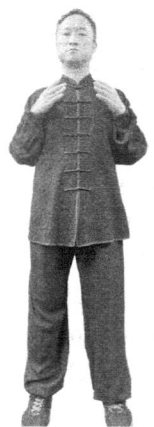

图 11
Fig. 11

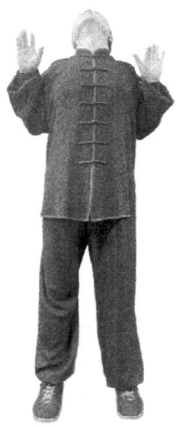

图 12
Fig. 12

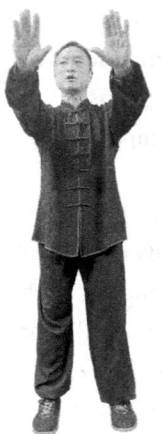

图 13
Fig. 13

（5）然后再落肘，夹肋，立掌，展肩扩胸，藏头缩项，推掌，口吐"呬"字音，如此重复练习六遍（图 13）。

【肌骨特征】

（1）夹肋时，两上臂要贴合身体，呈垂直姿势。

（2）展肩扩胸，藏头缩项时，不能耸肩。

（3）两膝缓缓伸直的同时，屈肘、两掌缓缓收拢至胸前约 10 厘米，与肩同高。

(5) Then, lower your elbows, tuck them by your ribs, position your hands with palms facing each other, expand your chest, tuck your head in, and push your palms forward, exhaling with the sound "Si". Repeat this practice six times (Fig. 13).

[Musculoskeletal Characteristics]

(1) When tucking your elbows by your ribs, ensure that your upper arms are close to your body in a vertical position.

(2) Expanding the shoulders and chest and tucking in the head and neck, you should avoid shrugging the shoulders.

(3) As you slowly straighten your knees, bend your elbows, and gradually move your palms together to a point about 10 cm in front of your chest, at shoulder height.

[Health Cultivation Elements]

The exercise associated with the "Si" Sound corresponds to the Lungs among the five internal organs. The lungs are connected with the autumn season, and exhaling during autumn helps to gather and moisten the lungs. Practicing more during autumn has the effect of regulating the flow of Qi, clearing the lungs of turbid Qi, and balancing lung function. This exercise method focuses on training the meridians and tendons of the neck, back, shoulders, and upper arms.

It can be utilized for the prevention and rehabilitation of conditions such as fever due to external pathogenic factors, dry cough without phlegm, dryness of the mouth and nose, and cracked skin. Additionally, it can serve as a traditional guiding method for conditions such as cervical spondylosis, myofascial pain syndrome in the back, and periarthritis of the shoulder.

【养生要素】

"呬"字功，与五脏之肺脏相应，肺与秋气相通，秋呬定收金肺润。秋季多练，具有通调气机、泻肺脏浊气、调理肺脏功能的作用。此功法动作着重锻炼颈项部、背部、肩部、上臂部的经筋。

可用于外感发热、干咳无痰、口鼻干燥、皮肤干裂等疾病的防治和康复。也可作为颈椎病、背部筋膜炎、肩关节周围炎等病症的传统导引方法。

第五式 "吹" 字 诀
Five "Chui" Zijue

扫码看视频

[Pronunciation and Mouth Shape]

The sound "Chui" (pronounced " 炊 ", flat tone) is a labial sound. When making the sound and exhaling, retract the tongue and

【发音与口型】

"吹"字音"chuī"（读炊，音平），属唇音。发声吐气时，舌体、嘴角后引，槽牙相对，两唇向两侧拉开收紧，气从喉出后，从舌两边绕舌下，经唇间缓缓呼出体外。

【动作描述】

接上式，两掌前推，然后松腕伸掌，变成掌心向下，两臂向左右分开，经侧平举向后划弧形，再下落至两掌心轻贴腰部；两膝下蹲，同时口吐"吹"字，两掌下滑，前摆，屈肘提臂于肚脐前成抱球姿势；两膝缓缓伸直，同时两掌慢慢收回至腹部，指尖斜向下，虎口相对；两掌沿带脉向后摩运至后腰部，然后再下滑，前摆，口吐"吹"字，如此重复练习六遍。

【分步练习】

（1）接上式。

（2）两掌前推，然后松腕伸掌，变成掌心向下，两臂向左右分开，经侧平

pull back the corners of the mouth, keeping the teeth aligned. Tighten and draw the lips to both sides, and as the breath exits the throat, let it gently pass around the sides of the tongue and out through the lips.

[Description of the Movement]

Continuing from the previous posture, push both palms forward, then relax the wrists and extend the palms, turning them to face downward. Open your arms to the sides, moving them horizontally and then backward in an arc, finally lowering them until your palms lightly touch your waist. As you squat down, exhale with the sound "Chui", letting your palms slide down, swing forward, and bend your elbows, raising your arms in front of your navel to form a ball-holding posture. Slowly straighten your knees while gradually bringing your palms back to the abdomen with fingertips pointing diagonally downward and the first web space of hands facing each other. Move your palms along the belt meridian to the lower back, then slide them down, swing forward, exhaling with the sound "Chui". Repeat this practice six times.

[Step-by-Step Practice]

(1) Continuing from the previous posture.

(2) Push both palms forward, then relax the wrists and extend the palms, turning them to face downward. Open your arms to the

sides, moving them horizontally and then backward in an arc, finally lowering them until your palms lightly touch your waist (Fig. 14).

(3) Slightly bend your knees and squat down while exhaling with the sound "Chui". Let your palms slide down and swing forward, fingers naturally spreading and fingertips facing each other. Slowly raise them to form a ball-holding posture in front of the navel (Fig. 15).

(4) Slowly straighten your knees while gradually bringing your palms together in front of the navel, fingertips pointing diagonally downward and the first web space of hands facing each other.

(5) Move your palms along the belt meridian to the lower back, then slide them

举向后划弧形，再下落至两掌心轻贴腰部（图14）。

（3）两膝微屈下蹲，同时口吐"吹"字，两掌下滑，前摆，十指自然分开，指尖相对，缓缓举至肚脐前成抱球姿势（图15）；

（4）两膝缓缓伸直，同时两掌缓缓收拢至肚脐前，指尖斜向下，虎口相对；

（5）两掌沿带脉向后摩运至后腰部，然后再下

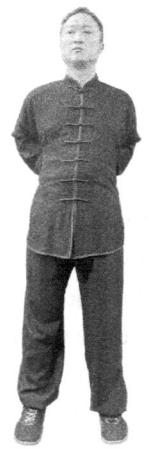

图 14
Fig. 14

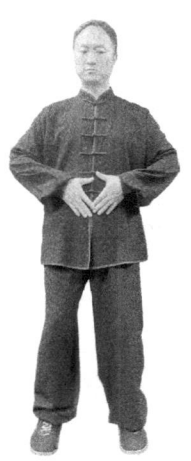

图 15
Fig. 15

滑,前摆,口吐"吹"字。如此重复练习六遍(图16)。

down, swing forward, and exhale with the sound "Chui". Repeat this practice six times (Fig. 16).

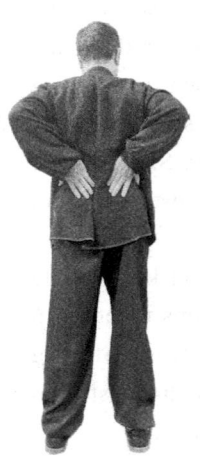

图 16
Fig. 16

【肌骨特征】

当屈肘提臂伸腕,于腹前形成抱球姿势时,髋膝关节要自然放松,两手掌相距约15厘米,肘关节形成的夹角约120°。

[Musculoskeletal Characteristics]

When you bend your elbows, raise your arms, and extend your wrists to form a ball-holding posture in front of your abdomen, and ensure that your hip and knee joints are naturally relaxed. Keep your hands approximately 15 cm apart, with the angle at your elbow joints around 120°.

【养生要素】

"吹"字功与五脏之肾脏相应,肾主冬,肾吹唯要坎中安。冬季多练,具有滋阴补阳、调理肾脏

[Health Cultivation Elements]

The "Chui" sound corresponds to the Kidneys among the five internal organs. The Kidneys govern Winter, and practicing this exercise in winter helps maintain balance in the kidney's functions. Frequent practice during winter nourishes Yin, supports Yang, and regulates kidney function. This exercise method focuses on training the meridians and tendons of the shoulders, upper arms, and waist.

It can be utilized for the prevention and rehabilitation of conditions such as lumbar and knee weakness, tidal fever and night sweats, dizziness, and tinnitus. Additionally, it can serve as a traditional guiding method for conditions such as periarthritis of the shoulder, myofascial inflammation of the lumbar and abdominal regions, and chronic lower back pain.

第六式 "嘻" 字诀
Six "Xi" Zijue

扫码看视频

[Pronunciation and Mouth Shape]

The sound "Xi" (pronounced " 希 ", flat tone) is a dental sound. When making the sound and exhaling, slightly open your lips and teeth, lightly press the tip of your tongue against the lower teeth, pull the corners of your mouth back slightly and upward, gently close the molars, and exhale so that the breath passes through the gaps between the molars and exits the body.

【动作描述】

接上式,两掌自然下落于体前,内旋,掌背相对,掌心向外,指尖向下,目视两掌。两膝缓缓伸直,同时提肘带手,经体前上提至胸,两手继续上提至面前,分掌、外开、上举,两臂呈弧形,掌心斜向上,目视前上方;屈肘。两手经面前收至胸前,两手与肩同高,指尖相对,掌心向下,目视前下方;屈膝下蹲,同时口吐"嘻"字,两掌缓缓下按至肚脐前;两掌继续向下,向左右外分至左右胯旁约15厘米处,掌心向外,指尖向下;两掌掌背相对,掌心向外,指尖向下,目视两掌;然后再上提,下按,口吐"嘻"字。如此重复练习六遍。

【分步练习】

(1)接上式。

[Description of the Movement]

Continuing from the previous posture, let your palms naturally fall in front of your body, rotate them inward so the backs of your hands face each other, palms facing outward, and fingertips pointing downward. Look at your palms. As you slowly straighten your knees, lift your elbows, moving your hands up in front of your body to chest level, then continue raising your hands in front of your face, separating and opening them outward and upward until your arms form an arc with palms slanted upward. Look slightly upward. Bend your elbows, bringing your hands back down in front of your face to chest level, with your hands at shoulder height, fingertips facing each other, and palms facing downward. Look slightly downward. As you squat down, exhale with the sound "Xi", and slowly press your palms down to in front of your navel. Continue moving your palms downward and outward to about 15 cm away from your hips, palms facing outward, and fingertips pointing downward. Rotate your hands so that the backs of your hands face each other, palms facing outward, and fingertips pointing downward. Look at your palms. Then, lift your hands up again and press down, exhaling with the sound "Xi". Repeat this practice six times.

[Step-by-Step Practice]

(1) Continuing from the previous

posture.

(2) Let your palms naturally fall in front of your body, rotating them inward so the backs of your hands face each other, palms facing outward, and fingertips pointing downward. Look at your palms (Fig. 17).

(3) As you slowly straighten your knees, lift your elbows and hands, bringing them up in front of your body to chest level. Continue raising your hands in front of your face, separating and opening them outward and upward until your arms form an arc with palms slanted upward. Look slightly upward (Fig. 18).

(4) Move your hands back down in front of your face to chest level, with your hands at shoulder height, fingertips facing each other, and palms facing downward.

（2）两掌自然下落于体前，内旋，掌背相对，掌心向外，指尖向下，目视两掌（图17）。

（3）两膝缓缓伸直，同时提肘带手，经体前上提至胸，两手继续上提至面前，分掌、外开，上举，两臂呈弧形，掌心斜向上，目视前上方（图18）。

（4）两手经面前收拢至胸前，两手与肩同高，指尖相对，掌心向下，目视前下方；屈膝下蹲，同

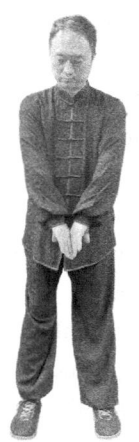

图 17
Fig. 17

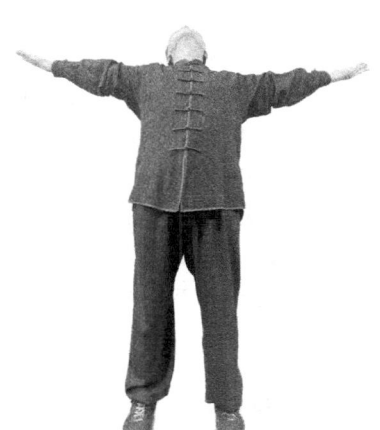

图 18
Fig. 18

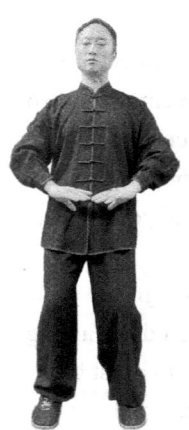

图 19
Fig. 19

时口吐"嘻"字，两掌缓缓下按至肚脐前（图19）。

（5）两掌继续向下，向左右外分至左右胯旁约15厘米处，掌心向外，指尖向下。

（6）两掌收至体前，掌背相对，掌心向外，指尖向下，目视两掌；然后再上提，下按，口吐"嘻"字。如此重复练习六遍。

【肌骨特征】

（1）练习时，沉肩、松肘，上肢运动要缓慢、

Look slightly downward. As you squat down, exhale with the sound "Xi", and slowly press your palms down to in front of your navel (Fig. 19).

(5) Continue moving your palms downward and outward to about 15 cm away from your hips, palms facing outward, and fingertips pointing downward.

(6) Move your palms back in front of your body with the backs of your hands facing each other, palms facing outward, and fingertips pointing downward. Look at your palms. Then, lift your hands up again and press down, exhaling with the sound "Xi". Repeat this practice six times.

[Musculoskeletal Characteristics]

(1) Keep your shoulders relaxed, elbows loose, and upper body movements

slow, gentle, and natural.

(2) Pressing down with both palms, you should focus your mind.

(3) Keep both feet still, maintain a stable center of gravity, raise both arms to about a 45° angle above shoulder level, and look slightly upward.

[Health Cultivation Elements]

The exercise associated with the character "Xi" corresponds to the triple energizer, which governs the transformation of Qi in the body, regulating the flow of Qi throughout the body's meridians. It can be practiced in all four seasons. This exercise method has the effect of clearing the triple energizer meridian, regulating the upper, middle, and lower burners (triple energizer), and promoting the smooth flow of Qi throughout the body. It focuses on training the meridians and tendons of the shoulders, upper arms, and wrists.

It can be utilized for the prevention and rehabilitation of conditions such as dizziness, tinnitus, chest and abdominal stuffiness, and difficulty urinating. Additionally, it can serve as a traditional guiding method for conditions such as cervical spondylosis, myofascial inflammation in the neck and back, and periarthritis of the shoulder.

柔和，变换动作要自然。

（2）下按两掌，意念集中。

（3）两脚不动，重心要稳，两臂上举至斜上方约45°，目视前上方。

【养生要素】

"嘻"字功与三焦相对应，主人体气化，通调全身气脉，四季皆可练。具有疏通少阳经，调理上、中、下三焦，畅通全身气机的作用。此功法动作着重锻炼肩部、上臂、腕部的经筋。

可用于眩晕、耳鸣、胸腹胀闷、小便不利等疾病的防治和康复。也可作为颈椎病、项背部筋膜炎、肩关节周围炎等病症的传统导引方法。

收　　势
Closing Posture

接上式，两手外旋，转掌心向内，缓缓收回，虎口交叉相握，轻抚肚脐，同时，两膝缓缓伸直，目视前下方，静养片刻；两掌以肚脐为中心揉腹，顺时针六圈，逆时针六圈，两掌松开，两臂自然下垂于体侧，中指贴于裤缝，目视前下方（图20，图21）。

Continuing from the previous posture, rotate both hands outward, turning your palms inward, and slowly bring them back, crossing your first web space of hands and gently resting your hands over your navel. At the same time, slowly straighten your knees and look downward, pausing for a moment to rest. Rub your abdomen with both palms, moving in a clockwise circle around the navel six times, then counterclockwise six times. Release your hands, allowing your arms to naturally hang at your sides, with your middle fingers touching the seams of your pants. Look slightly downward (Fig. 20, Fig. 21).

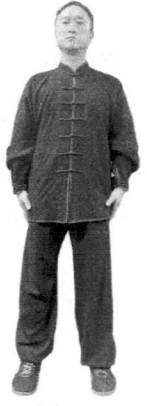

图 20
Fig. 20

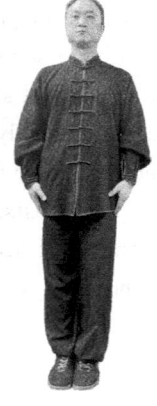

图 21
Fig. 21

第五章 常见病的防治

Chapter 5 Prevention and Treatment of Common Diseases

第一节 慢性阻塞性肺疾病
Section 1　Chronic Obstructive Pulmonary Disease

1. 医说析疑

慢性阻塞性肺疾病（COPD）是一种以呼吸困难、咳嗽、胸闷、喘息、疲劳为主要临床表现的慢性呼吸系统疾病。患病人群以老年人为主，随着空气污染的严重、人口老龄化加剧等因素的增加，慢性阻塞性肺疾病发病率呈现高发态势，且有越来越年轻化的趋势，更常见于吸烟和既往吸烟者。慢阻肺是一种无法治愈的慢性气道疾病，会逐渐侵蚀患者的肺功能，因此，有个可怕的外号，叫"沉默的杀手"。患病人群最大的困扰就是"咳痰喘"，早期会出现劳作时气短，随着病情进展、肺功能下降，平常生活中轻微的活动、正常走路，甚至休息时也会明显感觉气短、胸闷，需要大口呼吸，严重影响

1. Medical Theories Explained

Chronic Obstructive Pulmonary Disease (COPD) is a chronic respiratory disease characterized primarily by shortness of breath, coughing, chest tightness, wheezing, and fatigue. The majority of those affected are elderly, but with increasing air pollution and an aging population, the incidence of COPD is rising and affecting younger individuals, particularly smokers and former smokers. COPD is an incurable chronic airway disease that progressively deteriorates lung function, earning it the ominous nickname "the silent killer". The main issues for sufferers are "coughing, phlegm, and wheezing". Early symptoms include shortness of breath during physical activity, and as the disease progresses and lung function declines, even mild activities, normal walking, or resting can cause significant shortness of breath and chest tightness, necessitating deep breaths and severely impacting the quality of life. This disease causes continuous coughing throughout the year with excessive phlegm, and symptoms worsen in autumn and winter. Patients may experience shortness of breath and severe wheezing, akin to bellows, even after a few steps or climbing stairs. Moreover, long-term smoking habits and exposure to polluted air containing harmful gases or particles can trigger oxidative stress and inflammatory responses in the airways, contributing to the development of COPD. The lack of proper exercise, which fails to enhance physical and respiratory endurance, is also a significant factor in the onset and progression of COPD. Additionally, as people age, particularly elderly patients, their cardiopulmonary function and physical capacity decline noticeably. Due to slow metabolism, a monotonous diet, and decreased immunity, they are more prone to respiratory infections, accelerating the disease's progression. In severe cases, COPD can lead to chronic pulmonary heart disease, respiratory failure, and heart failure, posing a threat to the patient's life. Clinical treatments include oxygen therapy, bronchodilators, corticosteroids, and rehabilitation treatments such as breathing exercises and physical training.

As for stable COPD patients, the primary issue is a deficiency, particularly

患者的生活质量。这种疾病让患者一年到头咳个不停，痰还特别多，一到秋冬季节，症状更是严重，表现为上楼、走几步就气短、喘不上气，喘得就像拉风箱一样。再者，长期吸烟的不良习惯及暴露在有害气体或颗粒的污染空气中，也会引起气道氧化应激、炎症反应等多种途径参与慢阻肺发病。同时，缺乏合理的运动，无法提高运动能力和呼吸耐力，也是导致慢阻肺发生发展的重要原因。此外，随着年龄的增长，尤其是老年人患者，他们的心肺功能及运动能力明显下降，由于新陈代谢缓慢，饮食结构逐渐单一，免疫力进一步下降，更容易感染呼吸道疾病，加速疾病的恶化。严重者，会发展成慢性肺源性心脏病、呼吸衰竭和心力衰竭等，甚至危及患者生命。临床治疗上有氧疗、支气管扩张剂及糖皮质激素等药物，加以呼吸锻炼、运动训练等康复治疗。

稳定期COPD病人以本虚为主，主要表现为肺脾肾三脏亏虚，治疗上应以补虚为重。在六字诀呼吸法训练时进行"呬""呼""吹"字功训练，可改善肺脾肾功能。比如，在正常的饮食代谢情况下，通过"呼"字功训练可促进胃肠蠕动，使食物被充分吸收，从而使气血升化有源，四肢筋肉及脏腑得以濡养。另外，六字诀呼吸法训练还具有"调形"作用，即锻炼躯体的运动功能、协调四肢的柔韧性，从而加强身体的运动耐力和耐氧能力，改善患者的生活质量。

2. 防治方案

（1）改变生活中的不良习惯。患者吸烟的需要戒烟，避免被动吸烟、接触有害气体或颗粒，保持良好的生活习惯。加强锻炼，预防呼吸道感染，接种流感疫苗、肺炎链球菌疫苗等实现预防。

（2）六字诀功法套路动作。练习整个套路动作，

involving the lungs, spleen, and kidneys. Therefore, the treatment should focus on addressing these deficiencies. The practice of "Si", "Hu", and "Chui" sounds, helps improve the functions of the lungs, spleen, and kidneys. For example, under normal dietary metabolism, practicing the "Hu" exercise can promote gastrointestinal peristalsis and ensure that food is fully absorbed, which promotes the transformation of Qi and blood, thereby nourishing the muscles, tendons, and internal organs. Additionally, the Liuzijue breathing exercises incorporate bodily movements, which have a "regulating form" effect. This means they help enhance physical movement functions and coordinate the flexibility of the limbs, thereby improving physical endurance and oxygen capacity. Consequently, these exercises can significantly enhance the quality of life for COPD patients.

2. Prevention and Treatment Plan

(1) Changing Unhealthy Habits in Daily Life. Patients who smoke should quit smoking and avoid passive smoking or exposure to harmful gases or particles, maintaining good lifestyle habits. They should engage in regular exercise to prevent respiratory infections and receive vaccinations such as the influenza vaccine and pneumococcal vaccine for prevention.

(2) Liuzijue Routine Movements. Practise the entire routine of movements, or

focus on repeating the fourth "Si" and the sixth "Xi" techniques, each technique repeated six times, twice a day.

3. The Secret to Practice

Relax the whole body, concentrate the mind, maintain steady breathing. Movements should be gentle and relaxed, coordinated with breathing and vocalization, ensuring anatural flow. Pay attention to the transition of Yin and Yang in each posture, promoting the natural expansion and relaxation of muscles and joints. Breathing should be even, fine, gentle, and long, inhaling through the nose and exhaling slowly after a brief pause following each inhalation. The action requirement of the "Xu" exercise includes drawing the corners of the mouth backward, it is similar to the effect of pursed-lip breathing, it can alleviate the decrease in inspiratory airflow pressure, increase the internal pressure of small airways, promote the expulsion of residual air in the lungs, enhance alveolar ventilation, and thereby improve pulmonary microcirculation.

4. Points to Note

When starting the exercise, it's important to master correct pronunciation and control the volume, ensuring it's audible to yourself, and employing abdominal breathing and pursed-lip breathing. Each movement should be gentle and relaxed,

或者侧重反复练习第四式"呬"字诀,第六式"嘻"字诀,每个字诀重复练习六遍,每天2次。

3. 习练秘诀

全身放松、精神集中、呼吸平稳,动作要松柔舒缓,配合呼吸、吐音协调自然地去练套路动作,注意每式动作的阴阳转换,促使身体肌肉关节的膨胀然后放松自然的转换。呼吸要求做到"匀、细、柔、长",吸气时经鼻,每次吸气后不要忙于呼出,宜稍屏片刻,再徐徐呼出。"嘘"字诀的动作要求有嘴角后引,与缩唇呼吸的作用相似,可以缓解吸气气流压力下降,使小气道内压升高,促进肺部残气量的排出,增加肺泡通气量,从而改善肺微循环。

4. 注意事项

在开始锻炼时,要掌握正确的发音方式;控制音量,以自己耳朵能听见的音量为度;采用腹式呼吸、缩唇呼吸;每个动作要松柔舒缓;缓慢地增加运动次数，时间不宜过长。此外，锻炼总量要根据自身情况，逐渐进行增减。在锻炼的过程中会出现四肢关节处微微酸痛，这属于正常情况。

gradually increasing the number of repetitions without overextending the duration. Additionally, the overall exercise intensity should be adjusted according to individual condition, gradually increasing or decreasing as needed. It's normal to experience slight soreness in the joints of the limbs in the course of practice.

第二节　支气管哮喘
Section 2　Bronchial Asthma

1. 医说析疑

支气管哮喘（简称哮喘）是最常见的慢性呼吸系统疾病，可累及各个年龄段和任何种族的人群，以青壮年和儿童居多，一年四季可发作，但以春冬季发作为多见。这种疾病影响全球数亿人，具有间歇性和反复发作的特点，是一种气道慢性非特异性炎症疾病，常伴有广泛且多变的气流阻塞，此种炎症常导致反复发作的喘鸣、气短、胸闷和咳嗽等症状，易发于夜间或凌晨。发病原因复杂且多样化，且尚

1. Medical Theories Explained

Asthma, commonly referred to as bronchial asthma, is the most prevalent chronic respiratory disease, affecting individuals of all ages and ethnicities, with a higher incidence among young adults and children. It can occur throughout the year, although exacerbations are more common in spring and winter. This condition affects hundreds of millions of people worldwide and is characterized by intermittent and recurrent symptoms. Asthma is a chronic non-specific inflammatory airway disease often accompanied by widespread and variable airflow obstruction. This inflammation frequently leads to recurrent wheezing, shortness of breath, chest tightness, and coughing, which often occur at night or early in the morning. The causes of asthma are complex and diverse, and not entirely understood. It is currently believed to result from a combination of genetic and environmental factors, such as exposure to allergens, chemicals, air pollution, climate change, active and passive smoking, etc. The disease is prone to bacterial infections, and severe asthma can lead to pulmonary edema and even life-threatening situations. Asthma is a chronic disease that is considered manageable but not curable. Nowadays, it mainly requires a comprehensive treatment plan that includes medication, lifestyle adjustments, and avoidance of triggers. Drug therapy mainly includes anti-inflammatory drugs (such as corticosteroids), bronchodilators (such as albuterol inhalers), specific immunotherapy, and traditional Chinese medicine treatment, etc. Prevention and long-term control are key to preventing asthma attacks.

Based on clinical presentations, asthma can be classified into acute exacerbation phase, chronic persistent phase, and clinical control phase. Acute exacerbation of asthma refers to sudden onset or exacerbation of symptoms such as wheezing, shortness of breath, coughing, and chest tightness, characterized by decreased expiratory flow rates. It is often triggered by exposure to allergens, irritants, or respiratory infections.

不完全清楚，目前认为是遗传和环境因素（如接触过敏原、化学物质，空气污染、气候变化、主动和被动吸烟等）共同作用的结果。该病容易并发细菌感染，严重哮喘可致肺水肿，甚至危及生命。哮喘是慢性疾病，目前认为可控制，但不能治愈。目前主要采用包括药物治疗、生活方式调整和避免触发因素的综合治疗方案。药物治疗主要包括抗气道炎症的药物（如糖皮质激素等）、支气管扩张药（如沙丁胺醇气雾剂等）、特异免疫治疗和中医药治疗等。预防和长期控制是阻止哮喘发作的关键。

根据临床表现，哮喘可分为急性发作期、慢性持续期和临床控制期。哮喘急性发作是指喘息、气促、咳嗽、胸闷等症状突然发生，或原有症状加重，并以呼气流量降低为其特征，常因接触过敏原、刺激物或呼吸道感染诱发。其治疗的目的在于尽快缓解症状、解除气流受限和改善低氧血症，同时还需要制定长期治疗方案以预防再次急性发作。慢性持续期是指每周均不同频度和（或）不同程度地出现喘息、气促、胸闷、咳嗽等症状。其治疗的目的是尽可能避免接触过敏原或其他非特异刺激，这是防治哮喘最有效的方法。临床控制期是指患者无喘息、气促、胸闷、咳嗽等症状4周以上，1年内无急性发作，肺功能正常。其目标是达到良好的症状控制并维持正常活动水平，最大程度降低急性发作、固定性气流受限和药物不良反应的未来风险。各治疗级别方案中都应该按需使用缓解药物（快速支气管扩张剂）以迅速缓解症状，规律使用控制药物（吸入糖皮质激素）以维持症状的控制。

2. 防治方案

（1）改变生活中的不良习惯。尽量避免已知的过敏原和非特异性刺激物，保持室内环境的清洁和湿

The treatment goals are to quickly relieve symptoms, relieve airflow obstruction, and improve hypoxemia. Long-term treatment plans are also needed to prevent future acute exacerbations. The chronic persistent phase involves symptoms such as wheezing, shortness of breath, chest tightness, and coughing occurring at different frequencies and/or intensities each week. The treatment objective is to avoid, to the utmost extent, allergens, or other nonspecific stimuli, which is the most effective method for preventing and treating asthma. The clinical control phase refers to a period of at least 4 weeks without symptoms such as wheezing, shortness of breath, chest tightness, or coughing, and no acute exacerbations within a year, with normal lung function. The goal is to achieve good symptom control, maintain normal activity levels, minimize the future risks of acute exacerbations, fixed airflow obstruction, and adverse drug reactions. Relief medications (quick-acting bronchodilators) should be used as needed in all treatment regimens to rapidly relieve symptoms, while controller medications (inhaled corticosteroids) should be used regularly to maintain symptom control.

2. Prevention and Treatment Plan

(1) Changing Unhealthy Habits in Daily Life. Try to avoid known allergens and nonspecific irritants, maintain indoor cleanliness and moderate humidity levels,

engage in regular exercise while avoiding sudden strenuous activity, receive flu and pneumococcal vaccines to reduce the risk of respiratory infections, maintain a healthy lifestyle, undergo regular check-ups and treatments, and self-monitor condition.

(2) Liuzijue Routine Movements. Practice the entire routine of movements repeatedly or focus on repeatedly practicing of the first posture "Xu", the fourth posture "Si", and the fifth posture "Chui", each posture repeated six times, twice a day.

3. The Secret to Practice

Relax the whole body, concentrate the mind, maintain steady breathing. Movements should be gentle and relaxed, coordinated with breathing and vocalization, ensuring anatural flow. Pay attention to the transition of Yin and Yang in each posture, promoting the natural expansion and relaxation of muscles and joints. Breathing should be even, fine, gentle, and long, inhaling through the nose and exhaling slowly after a brief pause following each inhalation. Asthma is easily triggered in spring and winter. Therefore, it is advisable to focus on practicing the corresponding sounds: "Xu" for spring and "Chui" for winter. Following the sequence of the Five Elements, "Xu" corresponds to the Liver, associated with Wood and spring. Thus, practicing "Xu" can

功能的作用。"吹"与肾相对应,肾主水,相应于冬,多锻炼"吹"字功,肾具有纳气的功能。运用腹式呼吸,会使气息流畅,产生柔和的内脏按摩作用,从而改善内脏功能。

4. 注意事项

在开始锻炼时,要掌握正确的发音方式;控制音量,以自己耳朵能听见的音量为度;采用腹式呼吸、缩唇呼吸;每个动作要松柔舒缓;缓慢地增加运动次数,时间不宜过长。此外,锻炼总量要根据自身情况,逐渐进行增减。在锻炼的过程中会出现四肢关节处微微酸痛,这属于正常情况。

help regulate Liver function. "Chui" corresponds to the Kidneys, associated with Water and winter. Practicing "Chui" can help improve Kidneys function. Employing abdominal breathing facilitates smooth airflow and gentle internal organs massage, enhancing visceral function.

4. Points to Note

When starting the exercise, it's important to master correct pronunciation and control the volume, ensuring it's audible to yourself, and employing abdominal breathing and lip contraction breathing. Each movement should be gentle and relaxed, gradually increasing the number of repetitions without overextending the duration. Additionally, the overall exercise volume should be adjusted according to individual condition, gradually increasing or decreasing as needed. It's normal to experience slight soreness in the joints of the limbs in the course of practice.

第三节 咳 嗽
Section 3 Cough

1. 医说析疑

咳嗽是一种常见的临床症状,当咽喉部、支气

1. Medical Theories Explained

Coughing is a common clinical symptom, a defensive reflex triggered when the throat or bronchi are irritated by pollen, dust, or pathogens invading the respiratory tract to clear irritants, foreign objects, or secretions from the airway, ensuring safe breathing.

Coughing can be classified into acute, subacute, and chronic cough based on its duration. There are numerous causes of coughing. For instance, acute coughing is primarily caused by acute illnesses such as the common cold, influenza, pneumonia, asthma exacerbations, and respiratory tract foreign bodies. The most common cause of subacute coughing is post-infectious coughing. Allergic coughing, cough variant asthma, tracheitis, and gastroesophageal reflux disease are common causes of chronic coughing. Coughing can be very uncomfortable, ranging from mild symptoms like nasal itching, congestion, and difficulty breathing, to more severe symptoms such as fever, sleep disturbances, and respiratory distress, making individuals feel like their internal organs are being expelled. Coughing is also influenced by factors like diurnal rhythm, climate changes, body position changes, and irritants. For example, coughing frequency drops when sitting or standing, as the airways are less compressed, whereas lying down increases the difficulty of expelling foreign bodies or mucus due to airway collapse and surrounding organ

管受到花粉、灰尘刺激或病原体入侵时出现防御性反射，以清除呼吸道中的刺激物、异物或分泌物，从而让我们能保持安全呼吸。

咳嗽按照病程分为急性咳嗽、亚急性咳嗽和慢性咳嗽。引发咳嗽的原因非常多，比如，急性咳嗽主要是由于普通感冒、流感、肺炎、哮喘发作期及呼吸道异物等引起的急性疾病。亚急性咳嗽最常见的原因是感染后咳嗽。慢性咳嗽常见病因有过敏性咳嗽、咳嗽变异型哮喘、气管炎以及胃食管反流病等。咳嗽起来非常难受，轻的可能是鼻痒、鼻塞、呼吸不畅；严重起来伴随着发烧、睡不好、呼吸困难，感觉五脏六腑都要被咳出来了。咳嗽也与昼夜节律、气候变化、身体体位变化及刺激物有关，比如，站、坐位姿势时，呼吸道不受压迫，咳嗽发作频率减少；当卧位时，呼吸道偏塌陷，再加上周围器官和组织的压力，咳出异物或黏液的难度更大，得多咳几声来排出黏液。咳嗽除了病程长之外，也可能导致严重的并发症，甚至会引起支气管黏膜破裂、气胸等并发症。

2. 防治方案

（1）改变生活中的不良习惯。保持良好的个人卫生习惯，勤洗手，保证足够的营养及合理作息，适当参加体育锻炼，增强自身抵抗力。做好呼吸道隔离，保持室内空气新鲜，温度及湿度适宜，避免诱发阵发性咳嗽的因素。

（2）六字诀功法套路动作。练习整个套路动作，或者侧重反复练习第四式"呬"字诀，第五式"吹"字诀，第六式"嘻"字诀，每个字诀重复练习六遍，每天2次。

3. 习练秘诀

全身放松、精神集中、呼吸平稳，动作要松柔舒缓，配合呼吸、吐音协调自然地去练套路动作，注意每式动作的阴阳转换，促使身体肌肉关节的膨胀然后放松自然地转换。呼吸要求做到"匀、细、柔、

pressure, requiring several coughs to clear the mucus. Besides prolonging the course of illness, chronic coughing may lead to serious complications, including bronchial mucosal rupture and pneumothorax.

2. Prevention and Treatment Plan

(1) Changing Unhealthy Habits in Daily Life. Maintaining good personal hygiene habits such as frequent handwashing, ensuring adequate nutrition and a balanced lifestyle, participating in regular physical exercise, and enhancing one's immunity are essential. Implementing respiratory isolation measures, keeping indoor air freshness, and maintaining suitable temperature and humidity levels can help prevent factors that trigger paroxysmal coughing.

(2) Liu Zi Jue Routine Movements. Practise the entire routine of movements, or focus on repeatedly practicing the fourth posture "Si", the fifth posture "Chui", and the sixth posture "Xi", each posture repeated six times, twice a day.

3. The Secret to Practice

Relax the whole body, concentrate the mind, maintain steady breathing. Movements should be gentle and relaxed, coordinated with breathing and vocalization, ensuring anatural flow. Pay attention to the transition of Yin and Yang in each posture, promoting the natural expansion and relaxation of muscles and joints. Breathing should be even, fine, gentle, and long, inhaling through the nose and exhaling slowly after a brief pause following each inhalation. "Chui" corresponds to the Kidneys, which govern Water and correspond to winter. Practicing the "Chui" posture can enhance the Kidneys' ability to absorb Qi. Employing abdominal breathing facilitates smooth airflow and gentle internal organs massage, enhancing visceral function.

4. Points to Note

When starting the exercise, it's important to master correct pronunciation and control the volume, ensuring it's audible to yourself. Utilize abdominal breathing and pursed-lip breathing techniques. Each movement should be gentle and relaxed, gradually increasing repetitions without exceeding a lengthy duration. Additionally, adjust the exercise intensity based on personal condition, gradually increasing or decreasing as needed. It's normal to experience slight soreness in the joints of the limbs in the course of practice.

长",吸气时经鼻,每次吸气后不要忙于呼出,宜稍屏片刻,再徐徐呼出。"吹"与肾相对应,肾主水,相应于冬,多锻炼"吹"字功,肾具有纳气的功能。运用腹式呼吸,会使气息流畅,产生柔和的内脏按摩作用,从而改善内脏功能。

4. 注意事项

在开始锻炼时,要掌握正确的发音方式;控制音量,以自己能耳朵听见的音量为度;采用腹式呼吸、缩唇呼吸;每个动作要松柔舒缓;缓慢地增加运动次数,时间不宜过长。此外,锻炼总量要根据自身情况,逐渐进行增减。在锻炼的过程中会出现四肢关节处微微酸痛,这属于正常情况。

第四节 胸　闷
Section 4　Chest Tightness

1. 医说析疑

胸闷指患者自己能感受到胸部压迫感、紧缩、窒息或负重的不适感。这种感觉可能伴随着呼吸困难、疼痛、出汗和焦虑等。它可能是暂时的，也可能持续一段时间，出现胸闷可能是体内器官的功能性表现，也可能是疾病发病前兆或临床表现，青中老年各年龄段都可发生。可分为功能性胸闷和病理性胸闷两种类型。功能性胸闷是指没有器质性病变的胸闷，是指受周围环境和个人精神状态影响，自觉胸闷不适。例如，工作、居住环境长期密闭，或者抑郁状态、情绪不稳发生争吵，都可能会导致胸闷。此外，神经官能症如神经衰弱亦可导致功能性胸闷。病理性胸闷指的是器质性病变所致的胸闷，即由体内某器官病变引起。心血管、呼吸、消化系统疾病

1. Medical Theories Explained

Chest tightness, refers to the patient's perception of pressure, constriction, suffocation, or heaviness in the chest. This sensation may be accompanied by difficulty breathing, pain, sweating, and anxiety. It can be temporary or persist for a period of time and may indicate functional manifestations of organ dysfunction or be a precursor or clinical manifestation of disease. It can occur in people from youth to old age. Chest tightness can be classified into two types: functional and pathological. The former refers to the sensation of tightness without organic lesions in the chest, influenced by surrounding environments and personal mental states. For example, prolonged periods in closed work or living environments, or periods of depression and emotional instability leading to quarrels, may result in chest tightness. Additionally, conditions such as neurasthenia can also lead to functional chest tightness. The latter is caused by organic lesions within the body. Cardiovascular, respiratory, and digestive system diseases can all cause chest tightness. For example, cardiovascular diseases such as coronary heart disease, heart failure, rheumatic heart disease, and congenital heart disease can cause chest tightness. However, such chest tightness often has a history of underlying diseases and is accompanied by symptoms such as chest pain, palpitations, and shortness of breath. Severe cases or those in the middle and late stages often involve difficulty breathing and an inability to lie flat. Additionally, lung infections, chronic obstructive pulmonary diseases, and other respiratory conditions can also cause chest tightness. Some traumas, gastrointestinal diseases, as well as tumors in the neck and chest, can also lead to chest tightness. It not only poses challenges to work, study, and daily life but also burdens the body's health. Pathological chest tightness requires a thorough investigation of the underlying causes in order to treat the root cause.

2. Prevention and Treatment Plan

(1) Changing Unhealthy Habits in Daily Life. Maintaining a healthy mindset towards various circumstances, avoiding excessive worry, frustration, and anger, can help alleviate anxiety and stress. Adhering to a wholesome lifestyle by refraining from smoking and excessive alcohol consumption, as well as avoiding spicy foods, can contribute to overall well-being. Consistently engaging in moderate exercise

等均可引起胸闷。例如冠心病、心力衰竭、风湿性心脏病、先天性心脏病等心血管病均可引起胸闷，但此类胸闷既往多有基础疾病史，且伴有胸痛、心悸、气短，严重者或中后期多伴有呼吸困难，不能平卧等。此外，肺部感染、慢性阻塞性肺疾病等也是胸闷出现的原因。一些外伤、胃食管病以及颈、胸部的肿瘤亦可导致胸闷。病理性胸闷不但会给人们的工作、学习、生活造成困扰，也会给身体带来健康负担。这需要从源头查找病因，以便治病求本。

2. 防治方案

（1）改变生活中的不良习惯。正确对待各种事物，避免忧思郁怒，减少焦虑和压力。保持健康的生活方式，避免吸烟和过量饮酒，避免刺激性饮食。坚持合理运动，帮助改善心肺功能。

（2）六字诀功法套路动作。练习整个套路动作，或者侧重反复练习第一式"嘘"字诀，第二式"呵"字诀，第六式"嘻"字诀，每个字诀重复练习六遍，每天2次。

3. 习练秘诀

全身放松、精神集中、呼吸平稳，动作要松柔舒缓，配合呼吸、吐音协调自然地去练套路动作，注意每式动作的阴阳转换，促使身体肌肉关节的膨胀然后放松自然地转换。呼吸要求做到"匀、细、柔、长"，吸气时经鼻，每次吸气后不要忙于呼出，宜稍屏片刻，再徐徐呼出。按五行相生次序排列，"嘘"与肝相对应，肝属木，多锻炼"嘘"字功，具有疏通肝经、调畅气机、理气解郁的作用，可以改善肝气郁结证，使心情愉快。运用腹式呼吸，会使气息流畅，产生柔和的内脏按摩作用，从而改善内脏功能。

4. 注意事项

在开始锻炼时，要掌

can also aid in improving cardiovascular and pulmonary function.

(2) Liuzijue Routine Movements. Practise the entire routine of movements, or focus on repeating the first posture "Xu", the second posture "He", and the sixth posture "Xi", each repeated six times, twice a day.

3. The Secret to Practice

Relax the whole body, concentrate the mind, maintain steady breathing. Movements should be gentle and coordinated with breathing and vocalization, promoting a natural flow. Pay attention to the transition of Yin and Yang in each posture, encouraging the natural expansion and relaxation of muscles and joints. Breathing should be even, fine, gentle, and long, with inhalation through the nose followed by a slow exhalation after a brief pause. Following the sequence of the Five Elements, "Xu" corresponds to the Liver, which is associated with Wood. Practicing the "Xu" posture helps clear the Liver meridian, regulate Qi flow, and alleviate emotional stagnation, thus improving mood. Employing abdominal breathing facilitates smooth airflow and gentle internal organs massage, enhancing visceral function.

4. Points to Note

When starting the exercise, it's

important to master correct pronunciation and control the volume, making the sound heard by your own ears as a reference. Adopt abdominal breathing and pursed-lip breathing techniques. Each movement should be gentle and relaxed, gradually increasing the number of repetitions without extending the duration excessively. Additionally, the total exercise volume should be adjusted according to individual condition, gradually increasing or decreasing as needed. It's normal to experience slight soreness in the joints of the limbs in the course of practice.

第五节 心 悸
Section 5 Palpitations

1. Medical Theories Explained

Palpitations refer to a subjective sensation of abnormal heartbeat, usually manifested as rapid, intense, or irregular heartbeat, sometimes accompanied by the feeling of "skipped beats" or fluttering in the heart. Palpitations can be brief, sporadic, or prolonged, occurring suddenly during rest or during physical activity or intense emotions. It's a discomforting symptom; it could also indicate potential cardiac issues.

发生。它是一种让人不安的症状，也可能是潜在心脏问题的征兆。中老年患者可伴有心胸疼痛，喘息急促，汗出肢冷，甚则晕厥。心悸由多种原因引起，部分属于病理性，亦有不少是生理性。一般来说，健康人过度从事体力活动或情绪激动，如紧张、惊恐、焦虑以及大量吸烟、饮酒、饮浓茶、咖啡、缺乏睡眠、激烈运动时可感到明显心悸不适，这是一种生理现象。病理性心悸，临床上首先考虑心律失常所致，一般持续时间较长、不能自行缓解。此外，还包括心脏疾病、心理因素、药物作用、甲状腺功能亢进、贫血、感染等其他原因。频繁心悸对身体不利，轻微的会出现注意力不能集中，情绪不稳定，夜间入睡困难、多梦等，严重的可以引起血液循环失常，导致重要脏器供血不足，出现头晕、胸闷、乏力、心律失常。临床上心律失常变化往往比较迅速，严重的会导致猝死，需要及时就医。

In middle-aged and elderly patients, palpitations may be accompanied by chest pain, shortness of breath, sweating, and even syncope. Palpitations can be caused by various factors, some of which are pathological and others physiological. Generally, healthy individuals may experience palpitations due to excessive physical activity or emotional change such as nervousness, panic, anxiety, and smoking, alcohol consumption, caffeine intake, lack of sleep, or intense exercise, which are considered physiological responses. Pathological palpitations are clinically attributed to arrhythmias, which typically last longer and do not resolve on their own. Other causes include heart disease, psychological factors, medication effects, hyperthyroidism, anemia, infections, and more. Frequent palpitations can have detrimental effects on the body. Mild symptoms may include difficulty concentrating, mood swings, difficulty falling asleep, and vivid dreams, while severe cases can lead to disturbances in blood circulation, resulting in dizziness, chest tightness, fatigue, and arrhythmias. Changes in heart rhythm can occur rapidly, and severe cases may lead to sudden death, necessitating prompt medical attention.

2. Prevention and Treatment Plan

(1) Changing Unhealthy Habits in Daily Life. Maintain a healthy lifestyle by avoiding excessive fatigue, balancing your diet, engaging in moderate exercise, and getting sufficient sleep. Minimize intake of caffeine and nicotine, quit smoking, and limit alcohol consumption. Avoid emotional stress and excessive worrying to reduce anxiety and stress.

(2) Liuzijue Routine Movements. Practice the entire routine of movements, or focus on repeating the second posture "He", and the sixth posture "Xi", each posture repeated six times, twice a day.

3. The Secret to Practice

Relax the whole body, concentrate the mind, and maintain steady breathing. Perform movements gently and smoothly, coordinating with the breath and natural exhalation of sounds. Pay attention to the transformation of Yin and Yang in each posture, promoting the natural expansion and relaxation of muscles and joints. The breathing should be even, fine, soft, and long, inhaling through the nose and exhaling slowly after a brief pause. Following the sequence of the Five Elements, "He" corresponds to the Heart, which belongs to the Fire element and governs the blood vessels. Practicing "He" exercises can regulate the Heart meridian and improve

2. 防治方案

（1）改变生活中的不良习惯。保持健康的生活方式，避免过度疲劳，均衡饮食、适度锻炼和充分睡眠。避免摄入过多咖啡因和尼古丁、戒烟、忌酒。避免情志刺激以及思虑过度，减少焦虑和压力。

（2）六字诀功法套路动作。练习整个套路动作，或者侧重反复练习第二式"呵"字诀，第六式"嘻"字诀，每个字诀重复练习六遍，每天2次。

3. 习练秘诀

全身放松、精神集中、呼吸平稳，动作要松柔舒缓，配合呼吸、吐音协调自然地去练套路动作，注意每式动作的阴阳转换，促使身体肌肉关节的膨胀然后放松自然地转换。呼吸要求做到"匀、细、柔、长"，吸气时经鼻，每次吸气后不要忙于呼出，宜稍屏片刻，再徐徐呼出。按五行相生次序排列，"呵"与心相对应，心属火，主血脉，多锻炼"呵"字功，具有疏通心经、调理心脏功能的作用。"嘻"与三焦相对应，多锻炼"嘻"字功，具有调理三焦、畅通全身气机的作用。运用腹式呼吸，会使气息流畅，产生柔和的内脏按摩作用，从而改善内脏功能。

heart function. "Xi" corresponds to the triple energizer and practicing "Xi" exercises can regulate the triple energizer and promote the smooth flow of Qi throughout the body. Employing abdominal breathing facilitates smooth airflow and gentle internal organs massage, enhancing visceral function.

4. 注意事项

在开始锻炼时，要掌握正确的发音方式；控制音量，以自己耳朵能听见的音量为度；采用腹式呼吸、缩唇呼吸；每个动作要松柔舒缓；缓慢地增加运动次数，时间不宜过长。此外，锻炼总量要根据自身情况，逐渐进行增减。在锻炼的过程中会出现四肢关节处微微酸痛，这属于正常情况。

4. Points to Note

When starting to exercise, it's important to master correct pronunciation and control the volume, using the level that you can hear with your own ears as a guide. Adopt abdominal breathing and lip-pursed breathing. Each movement should be gentle and relaxed, gradually increasing the number of repetitions and avoiding overly long sessions. Additionally, adjust the total exercise volume according to your own condition, gradually increasing or decreasing as needed. It's normal to experience slight soreness in the joints of the limbs in the course of practice.

第六节　颈　椎　病
Section 6　Cervical Spondylosis

1. 医说析疑

颈椎病又称颈椎综合

1. Medical Theories Explained

Cervical spondylosis, also known as

cervical spondylopathy, refers to degenerative changes in the cervical intervertebral discs and secondary pathological changes in adjacent structures, involving surrounding tissues (such as nerves, blood vessels, spinal cord, etc.), and accompanied by a series of clinical syndromes corresponding to imaging changes. It is mainly manifested as neck and shoulder pain, dizziness, headache, numbness in the upper limbs, muscle atrophy, chest tightness, palpitations, and in severe cases, spasms in the lower limbs, difficulty walking, and even paralysis of the limbs, urinary and fecal disorders, and paralysis. Due to different specific types, the clinical manifestations, treatment methods, and prognosis also vary. Below is a detailed introduction to various types of cervical spondylosis.

(1) Neck type of cervical spondylosis. Neck type of cervical spondylosis (localized cervical spondylosis) refers to a series of symptoms such as neck and shoulder pain, limited mobility, and arm soreness and numbness caused by the straightening or reverse curvature of the cervical spine, intervertebral disc degeneration, osteophyte formation, and the inability of the cervical spine to reduce load. It is the most common and mildest type of cervical spondylosis. The symptoms are often mild and may be frequently overlooked clinically. If left untreated or if the neck type of cervical

征，是指颈椎间盘退行性改变及其继发的相邻结构病理改变，累及周围组织结构（神经、血管、脊髓等），并出现与影像学改变相应的一系列症状的临床综合征。它主要表现为颈肩痛、头晕头痛、上肢麻木、肌肉萎缩、胸闷、心慌，严重者双下肢痉挛、行走困难，甚至四肢麻痹、大小便障碍、瘫痪。因具体类型不同，其临床表现也是各异，治疗方式及预后也是不同的。下面具体介绍一下各个类型的颈椎病。

（1）颈型颈椎病。颈型颈椎病（局限性颈椎病）是指由于颈椎生理曲度变直或反弓、颈椎间盘退化、骨质增生、颈椎减重功能不能降低而出现的一系列颈肩部疼痛、活动不利、手臂酸麻胀痛等症状。颈型颈椎病是最多见的，也是症状较轻的一个类型。往往症状比较轻微，临床上可能经常会被忽视，如果颈型颈椎病迁延不愈，处理不当，非常容易发展成其他类型的颈椎病。随着社会压力的不断增加和电子产品的广泛使用，各行各业人群长期处于低头状态，又缺乏运动，近年来颈椎病的发病呈高态势，在青少年人群中患病率很高。门诊中经常碰到有年轻患者来就诊，询问自己颈部活动时颈椎会有咔咔响声，肩膀高低不平衡、身体歪了等不美观体态及不适症状。主要原因是长时间低头固定一个姿势牵拉斜方肌肌纤维，使其处于紧张、痉挛的状态，出现斜方肌一侧紧张挛缩导致颈肩部疼痛及两侧肩部不平衡的高低肩的体态表现。进一步发展会导致颈椎骨关节的位置变化，如出现骨质增生、生理曲度变直或反弓等结构改变，使颈椎结构和功能稳定受到不同程度的损害。

（2）神经根型颈椎病。此类型在各型颈椎病中发病率较高、临床多见，主要表现为与脊神经根分布区相一致的感觉、运动及反射障碍，表现为颈项部疼痛，向肩、臂、前臂及

spondylosis persists, it can easily progress to other types of cervical spondylosis. With increasing societal pressures and widespread use of electronic devices, individuals across various professions often maintain a prolonged forward-head posture and lack physical activity, in recent years, the incidence of cervical spondylosis has been on the rise, especially for the young people. In outpatient clinics, it is common to encounter young patients seeking treatment for symptoms such as cracking sounds in the neck during movement, uneven shoulders, body asymmetry, and increasing prominence of the hump. The main reason for this is the prolonged fixed posture of looking down, which causes traction on the fibers of the trapezius muscle, leading to tension and spasms, resulting in neck and shoulder pain and the uneven shoulder posture. This further leads to changes in the position of the cervical vertebral joints, such as osteophyte formation or changes in the physiological curvature. Consequently, the stability and function of the cervical spine are compromised to varying degrees.

(2) Nerve root type of cervical spondylotic. This type of cervical spondylosis is one of the most common types among all cervical spondylosis cases, characterized by sensory, motor, and reflex disorders consistent with the distribution of spinal nerve roots. Symptoms include neck pain

radiating to the shoulders, arms, forearms, and fingers, accompanied by weakness and numbness in the upper limbs, most often unilateral. Muscle weakness may occur due to nerve supply to the muscles. This condition is more common in middle-aged and elderly individuals, but in recent years, it has been increasingly observed in younger people. Even children as young as ten have reported symptoms such as neck pain, hand numbness, and discomfort. Positive findings in tests such as the foraminal compression test or the brachial plexus traction test, along with imaging evidence of corresponding nerve root compression, are consistent with clinical symptoms, which can lead to a diagnosis of nerve root type of cervical spondylosis. Younger individuals nowadays typically develop cervical spondylosis due to prolonged desk work or study, and prolonged use of smartphones in a forward head posture. Chronic poor neck posture leads to chronic strain on the cervical spine, gradually affecting the muscles, ligaments, and stability of the cervical joints. For instance, prolonged forward head posture increases the load on the cervical spine, particularly in the lower cervical segments, resulting in increased pressure on the intervertebral discs, which can easily cause disc herniation, leading to compression or irritation of the cervical nerve roots and gradually resulting in symptoms such as

手指放射，同时可伴上肢乏力及手指麻木，大多数单侧发作。神经支配肌肉，会引起肌肉乏力。本病好发于中老年人，近年来临床上碰到的发病人群越来越年轻化了，甚至有十多岁的孩子也出现了脖子痛，还有手麻、酸胀痛。通过检查椎间孔挤压试验或臂丛牵拉试验呈阳性，影像学显示相应神经根受压征象与临床症状相一致，可以诊断为神经根型颈椎病。现在的中青年基本上都是因为长期伏案工作或学习和长时间低头玩手机、用电脑等不良姿势引起的颈椎病。长期的不良颈椎姿势，演变成颈椎的慢性劳损，慢性期逐渐累及颈部肌肉、韧带及骨关节稳定性。比如，长时间的低头，使颈椎承重更大，越往下，下颈段承重功能体现得越明显，它的椎间盘受压也更明显，很容易造成椎间盘突出使颈神经根受压或刺激，逐渐引起上肢疼痛、麻木等根性症状。除了椎间盘源性之外，还有颈椎后方小关节的松动与移位及骨质增生、钩椎关节骨赘形成导致，病人常有不同程度的颈部活动障碍。颈椎骨关节面附着的很多肌肉、韧带一同劳损，可能影响颈椎的稳定性，颈部、肩部肌肉张力增高或痉挛，从而引起疼痛。颈椎不稳定、骨质增生及软组织的损伤对脊神经根造成刺激与压迫，与颈脊神经所支配的组织区域出现疼痛、麻木的根性症状。肌肉的劳损同样可以引起肩臂的疼痛、麻木，比如，斜角肌的紧张、痉挛会刺激神经，容易引起颈、胸、背、肩、臂部疼痛，出现手麻的症状，以及影响低头、转头、侧屈等动作。

（3）椎动脉型颈椎病。椎动脉型颈椎病常常因为脖子扭转后出现头晕、站立不稳、恶心、想吐的症状，其特点是发病突然，来势是凶猛的，突发性眼花，严重的会引起猝倒。猝倒是此类型的一个表现，但意识是清楚的。椎动脉因

upper limb pain and numbness. In addition to disc-related factors, patients often experience restricted cervical mobility dueto, laxity and displacement of the posterior facet joints of the cervical spine, osteophyte formation at the uncovertebral joints, and strain on many muscles and ligaments attached to the cervical facet joints can affect cervical stability. Increased tension or spasm in the neck and shoulder muscles may also lead to pain. Instability of the cervical spine, osteophyte formation, and soft tissue damage can irritate and compress the spinal nerve roots, causing pain and numbness in the regions supplied by the cervical spinal nerves. Muscle strain can also cause shoulder and arm pain and numbness. For example, tension or spasm of the trapezius muscle can stimulate nerves, resulting in symptoms such as pain in the neck, chest, back, shoulders, and arms, as well as numbness in the hands, and limitations in movements such as bending, turning, and tilting the head.

(3) Vertebral artery type of cervical spondylosis. Vertebrobasilar artery type of cervical spondylosis often manifests as dizziness, instability when standing, nausea, and vomiting after one twists the neck. Its hallmark is its sudden onset and severity, with sudden onset vertigo that can lead to fainting. Syncope is a manifestation of this type, but consciousness remains clear.

Vertebrobasilar artery type of cervical spondylosis occurs due to compression or irritation of the vertebral artery for various reasons, leading to insufficient blood supply to the vertebrobasilar artery, hence the name. This is a common condition among middle-aged and elderly individuals, with approximately 70% of cervical spondylosis patients experiencing involvement of the vertebral artery. Over 50% of individuals above fifty years old experiencing dizziness or headache are related to vertebral artery involvement caused by cervical spondylosis. In middle-aged and elderly patients, cervical segmental instability or narrowed intervertebral spaces can cause twisting and compression of the vertebral artery. Osteophyte formation can also directly compress the vertebral artery, leading to spasm and sudden changes in vertebral artery blood flow, resulting in symptoms of inadequate blood supply. Young patients who visit outpatient clinics often experience dizziness, weakness, nausea, and sometimes visual impairment or blurriness when turning, bending, or changing positions. Though they undergo examinations in neurology and otolaryngology departments, the cause of these discomforting symptoms cannot be determined. X-ray examinations often show no osteophyte formation, and the cervical spine is relatively stable. However, positive results in the vertebral

各种原因受到压迫或刺激而引起椎—基底动脉供血不足而诱发疾病，所以叫椎动脉型颈椎病。这是中老年人的常见病，颈椎病患者中约70%有椎动脉受累。五十岁以上头晕、头痛者，50%以上与颈椎病引起的椎—基底动脉受累有关。中老年患者发病原因主要是颈椎出现节段性不稳定、椎间隙狭窄，造成椎动脉扭曲并受到挤压；骨质增生的形成也可以直接压迫椎动脉，使椎动脉痉挛而出现椎动脉血流瞬间变化，导致供血不足而出现症状。而门诊中前来就诊的年轻患者常常转头、低头或变换体位时容易出现头晕、乏力、恶心、想吐，有时候还有视力下降或模糊。他们去了神经内科和耳鼻喉科做了检查后也确定不了是什么疾病导致的这些不适症状。X光片检查显示往往没有骨质增生，颈椎也相对较稳定，椎动脉扭曲试验阳性，低头仰头试验阳性，发病主要还是长时间低头工作、玩手机、用电脑和缺乏锻炼，导致颈部深层肌群的损伤，刺激椎动脉周围的交感神经纤维引起的。

（4）脊髓型颈椎病。这种病比较凶险，甚至可造成肢体瘫痪，致残率最高。严重的需要手术治疗，如果治疗不及时，脊髓的损伤是不可逆的。

除了外伤造成的，脊髓型颈椎病通常起病缓慢，以40～60岁的中年人为多。脊髓型颈椎病的发病及严重程度，往往和有无颈椎管狭窄有很大关系。颈椎骨质增生、韧带肥厚和椎间盘突出形成的椎管狭窄刺激和压迫脊髓是主要原因。X光片上显示椎体后缘骨质增生、椎管狭窄，MRI显示脊髓压迫。多数患者先出现一侧或双侧下肢麻木、沉重、踩棉花感，严重者逐渐出现步态不稳、行走困难，上下楼梯时需要借力。躯干部

artery torsion test and the head flexion-extension test indicate that the main cause of the condition is deep muscle damage in the neck due to prolonged periods of working with the head bent, using smartphones or computers, and lack of exercise, leading to stimulation of the sympathetic nerve fibers around the vertebral artery.

(4) Spinal cord type of cervical spondylosis. It is one of the most dangerous and severe types of cervical spondylosis, which can even cause limb paralysis. The disability rate is the highest for this type, and it often requires surgical treatment. If not treated promptly, the damage to the spinal cord is irreversible.

Apart from trauma-induced cases, spinal cord type of cervical spondylosis typically has a slow onset, mostly affecting middle-aged individuals between 40 and 60 years old. The onset and severity of spinal cord type of cervical spondylosis are often closely related to the presence of cervical spinal canal stenosis. The main causes are the stimulation and compression of the spinal cord due to cervical osteophyte formation, ligament hypertrophy, and intervertebral disc protrusion leading to spinal canal stenosis. X-rays show osteophyte formation at the posterior edge of the vertebrae and spinal canal stenosis, while MRI reveals spinal cord compression. Most patients initially experience numbness, heaviness, or a sensation of stepping on cotton in one or both lower limbs. Severe cases may develop gait instability and difficulty walking, requiring assistance in climbing stairs. Sensory abnormalities may also occur in the trunk, with patients feeling a belt-like sensation in the chest or abdomen, along with burning or cold sensations in the lower limbs. A small number of patients may experience urinary and bowel dysfunction, such as urinary frequency, urgency, incomplete emptying, incontinence, constipation, and sexual dysfunction. For early-stage central and anterior central vascular types, non-surgical therapy may be considered. However, if symptoms worsen over time or suddenly, or if non-surgical treatment is ineffective in relieving spinal cord damage, surgical intervention should be promptly pursued. In cases of acute progressive spinal cord injury confirmed by CT scans and contrast imaging, surgery should be performed as soon as possible.

(5) Sympathetic nervous type of cervical spondylosis. It is the most troublesome and complex type of cervical spondylosis because its symptoms are variable, leading to a higher rate of misdiagnosis and unclear treatment effects. Factors such as intervertebral disc degeneration, vertebral instability, muscle tension, and spasms around the cervical

也会出现感觉异常，患者常感觉在胸腹部或双下肢有如皮带样的捆绑感，同时下肢可有烧灼感、冰凉感。极少数患者出现排尿无力、尿频尿急尿不尽、尿失禁或尿潴留、大便秘结等排尿排便障碍，以及性功能减退。早期的中央型及前中央血管型患者可采用非手术疗法。对脊髓受到长期损害并症状日渐或突然加重，非手术疗法无效者，应及时采取手术治疗。对急性进行性脊髓损害，CT扫描及造影已经确诊者应尽快手术。

（5）交感神经型颈椎病。这种病是最麻烦、最复杂的颈椎病，因为其症状多变，误诊率比较大，治疗效果也不明显。由于椎间盘退化、椎体不稳定、肌肉紧张痉挛等因素导致颈椎周围交感神经末梢出现了刺激，然后产生了交感神经功能的紊乱。比如,胸锁乳突肌参与了颈椎大部分的活动,涉及头部侧屈、低头、左右旋转等功能。胸锁乳突肌的紧张痉挛会刺激交感神经、颈横神经、耳大神经、颈动脉出现症状。临床表现相较其他类型的颈椎病比较多,多数表现为交感神经兴奋症状,少数为交感神经抑制症状,且伴有椎动脉症状,X光片显示颈椎有骨质增生、退变或失稳,椎动脉造影阴性可作为辅助诊断。除了颈背部疼痛、麻木的症状之外,还有头部症状,表现出头痛、眩晕、偏头痛、睡眠障碍、注意力不集中、记忆力减退等;五官部症状,如眼胀、眼干、流泪、视物模糊、耳鸣、听力下降、鼻塞、口干、声带疲劳、咽部异物感等;胃肠道症状,如恶心、呕吐、腹胀、腹泻、消化不良等;心血管症状,如心悸、胸闷、心律失常、血压变化等。这类型的症状是反复发作、迁延难愈,非常折磨人的一类颈椎病。一般采用非手术治疗,症状严重者可考虑手术治疗。以上症状

spine can stimulate the sympathetic nerve endings, resulting in dysfunction of the sympathetic nervous system. For instance, the sternocleidomastoid muscle participates in most movements of the cervical spine, including lateral bending, flexion, and rotation. Tension and spasms in the sternocleidomastoid muscle can stimulate the sympathetic nerves, cervical plexus, auricular nerves, and carotid arteries, leading to symptoms. Clinical manifestations are more varied compared to other types of cervical spondylosis, with more presenting symptoms of sympathetic nervous system excitation and fewer showing symptoms of sympathetic nervous system inhibition, often accompanied by symptoms related to the vertebral artery. X-rays may reveal osteophyte formation, degeneration, or instability in the cervical spine, while negative vertebral artery angiography can serve as an auxiliary diagnostic tool. In addition to symptoms such as neck and back pain and numbness, other symptoms may include head symptoms: headache, dizziness, migraine, sleep disturbances, lack of concentration, and memory decline. Sensory symptoms: eye pain, dry eyes, tearing, blurred vision, tinnitus, hearing loss, nasal congestion, dry mouth, vocal fatigue, and throat discomfort. Gastrointestinal symptoms: nausea, vomiting, abdominal distension, diarrhea, and indigestion.

Cardiovascular symptoms: palpitations, chest tightness, arrhythmias, and changes in blood pressure. These symptoms often recur and are difficult to resolve, making this type of cervical spondylosis extremely distressing. Non-surgical treatments are generally used, but surgery may be considered for severe cases. These symptoms are often closely related to neck movements, worsening with factors such as prolonged desk work, prolonged use of mobile phones and computers, fatigue, as well as worsening during sitting or standing, and alleviating or disappearing after resting in a lying position.

2. Prevention and Treatment Plan

(1) Changing Unhealthy Habits in Daily Life. It's important to keep the neck warm, maintain a good sleeping posture, choose a pillow that is suitable in terms of firmness and height to ensure proper alignment of the neck, and prevent neck injuries. Additionally, strengthening exercises for the neck and shoulder muscles are beneficial, such as practicing specific exercises, swimming, playing badminton, basketball, and other sports activities.

(2) Liuzijue Routine Movements. Practise the entire routine of postures or focus on repeatedly practicing the first posture "Xu", the fourth posture "Si", and the sixth posture "Xi". Repeat each posture six times, twice a day.

每天 2 次。

3. 习练秘诀

全身放松、精神集中、呼吸平稳，动作要松柔舒缓，配合呼吸、吐音协调自然地去练套路动作，注意每式动作的阴阳转换，促使身体肌肉关节的膨胀然后放松自然转换。呼吸要求做到"匀、细、柔、长"，吸气时经鼻，每次吸气后不要忙于呼出，宜稍屏片刻，再徐徐呼出。"呬"字诀的动作要求夹肋、展肩扩胸、藏头缩项、不能耸肩。在吐"呬"字音时，伸展头颈部，同时扩展肩部、上肢，着重锻炼颈项部、背部、肩部、上臂部的经筋。

4. 注意事项

在开始锻炼时，要掌握正确的发音方式；控制音量，以自己耳朵能听见的音量为度；采用腹式呼吸、缩唇呼吸；每个动作要松柔舒缓；缓慢地增加运动次数，时间不宜过长。此外，锻炼总量要根据自身情况，逐渐进行增减。在锻炼的过程中会出现颈

3. The Secret to Practice

Relax the whole body, concentrate the mind, maintain steady breathing. Perform movements with gentleness and fluidity, coordinating with the breath and vocalization. Pay attention to the transition between Yin and Yang in each posture, encouraging the natural expansion and relaxation of muscles and joints. Breathe evenly, softly, and deeply, inhaling through the nose and exhaling slowly without haste, pausing briefly between breaths. In the "Si" posture, rib compression, shoulder expansion, chest opening, and maintaining a tucked chin without shrugging the shoulders are emphasized. When vocalizing the "Si" sound, extend the head and neck while simultaneously expanding the shoulders and upper limbs, focusing on strengthening the meridians and tendous of the neck, back, shoulders, and upper arms.

4. Points to Note

When starting the exercise, it's important to master the correct pronunciation and control the volume, using the level that you can hear with your ears as a guide. Additionally, adopt abdominal breathing and pursed-lip breathing techniques. Each movement should be gentle and relaxed, gradually increasing the number of repetitions and avoiding excessive duration. Furthermore, adjust the total exercise volume according to your own condition, gradually increasing or decreasing as needed. It's normal to experience slight soreness in the neck and limbs joints in the course of practice.

椎、四肢关节处微微酸痛，这属于正常情况。

第七节 腰 痛
Section 7　Lower Back Pain

1. Medical Theories Explained

Clinically encountered types of lower back pain often include acute lumbar sprain, chronic lumbar muscle strain, lumbar disc herniation, lumbar spinal stenosis, third lumbar transverse process syndrome, and postpartum lower back pain.

(1) Acute lumbar sprain. Commonly known as "throwing out the back" or "twisting the waist," Acute lumbar sprain often occurs in young and middle-aged adults, manual laborers, and individuals who lack regular physical exercises. It is frequently encountered in outpatient clinics, where patients present with severe lower back pain, movement of the lumbar spine in various directions is restricted, with forward bending and backward extension being particularly difficult. Patients may walk with a stooped posture, unable to straighten their

1. 医说析疑

临床上常遇到的腰痛可以分为以下几类：急性腰扭伤、慢性腰肌劳损、腰椎间盘突出症、第三腰椎横突综合征、腰椎管狭窄症产后腰痛。

（1）急性腰扭伤。俗称"闪腰""岔气"，多发生于青壮年、体力劳动者及平时缺乏体育锻炼者。在门诊非常多见，就诊的患者腰部疼痛难忍，腰椎各方向活动受限，前屈、后伸方向较为困难，得弯着腰走路、腰直不起来，咳嗽、大声说话、腹部用力时均可使疼痛加重，多用双手撑腰，借以防止因活动而发生更剧烈的疼痛，严重者身体弯向一侧不能动弹。多因腰部突然扭转、活动姿势不正确或搬抬重物时肌肉不配合、不协调，以及跌扑损伤造成的腰部肌肉、韧带、筋膜及小关节急性损伤所致。另外，经常发作急性腰扭伤后出现腰痛呈渐进加重，且伴有下肢疼痛、麻木、无力甚至大小便功能障碍者，需要特别重视，应及时就医，通过相关影像检查，确认是否为腰椎间盘突出症造成的神经损伤。急性腰扭伤若处理不当或治疗不及时，症状会迁延不愈，可演变成慢性腰肌劳损。

（2）慢性腰肌劳损。慢性腰肌劳损是腰部软组织，包括肌肉、筋膜等的慢性损伤，在劳损部位局部形成炎性改变，从而引起腰部隐痛、反复发作、

backs. Coughing, speaking loudly, or exerting abdominal pressure can exacerbate the pain. Many individuals find relief by supporting their lower back with their hands to prevent exacerbating the pain during movement. In severe cases, the body may be bent to one side and immobile. Acute lumbar sprain is often caused by sudden twisting of the waist, incorrect posture during movement, muscle coordination issues when lifting heavy objects, or falls resulting in acute injury to the muscles, ligaments, fascia, and small joints of the lumbar region. Moreover, individuals who frequently experience acute lumbar sprains followed by progressive aggravation of lower back pain, along with leg pain, numbness, weakness, or even dysfunction of bowel and bladder control, require special attention. Prompt medical attention and relevant imaging examinations are necessary, as these symptoms may indicate nerve damage caused by lumbar disc herniation. Improper management or delayed treatment of acute lumbar sprain can lead to prolonged symptoms and the development of chronic lumbar muscle strain.

(2) Chronic lumbar muscle strain. Chronic lumbar muscle strain refers to the chronic damage to the soft tissues in the lower back, including muscles and fascia, resulting in local inflammatory changes, leading to symptoms primarily characterized

by persistent, recurrent lower back pain that worsens after exertion, with a history of acute lumbar muscle strain in most cases. Clinically, the pain can vary in intensity and worsen after exertion, but alleviate with rest. Tender points may be localized to specific areas or dispersed throughout the lower back, with tenderness commonly found around the sacrospinalis, posterior iliac crest, sacrum, and lumbar transverse processes.

(3) Lumbar disc herniation. In addition to lower back pain, if there is also numbness in one or both legs, it may be a sign of lumbar disc herniation. Lumbar disc protrusion and lumbar disc herniation are two different concepts. In outpatient clinics, some patients bring their lumbar spine CT or MRI reports and ask the doctor, "The report shows that my lumbar disc is protruding, what should I do?" Clinically, "lumbar disc herniation" refers to the protrusion of the intervertebral disc pressing on the nerve, causing local inflammation and other reactions, resulting in corresponding symptoms and signs such as pain and numbness in the affected area. When this happens, we call it lumbar disc herniation. However, not all cases of disc protrusion lead to symptoms. In such cases, it's referred to simply as disc protrusion, indicating degenerative changes in the lumbar intervertebral disc and a high risk of

劳累后加重为主要表现的疾病，大多既往有急性腰扭伤史。临床特点是时轻时重，劳累后加重，休息后减轻。痛点可局限于某个部位，也可散布于整个腰部。腰部有压痛，多在骶棘肌处、髂骨后部、骶骨后骶棘肌止点处或腰椎横突处。

（3）腰椎间盘突出症。除了腰部疼痛，如果伴有一侧、两侧下肢麻木感，这可能是腰椎间盘突出症的表现。腰椎间盘突出和腰椎间盘突出症是两个不同的概念，门诊常有些患者拿着腰椎的CT或磁共振检查报告问医生"报告显示我腰椎间盘突出了，该怎么办？"临床上说的"腰椎间盘突出症"，指的是椎间盘突出压迫到神经，引起局部的炎症等反应，进而出现相应区域的疼痛和麻木等症状和体征时，我们就说这是椎间盘突出症。椎间盘突出后并不一定会出现症状，这种情况还只能叫椎间盘突出，说明腰椎间盘已经退行性改变，发病风险很高，很可能由于简单的弯腰下蹲、搬重物、用力咳嗽、久坐等情况导致髓核突出压迫神经，形成腰椎间盘突出症。

腰椎间盘突出症常常是在椎间盘退变的基础上产生的，病理上主要是因为腰椎间盘各部分（髓核、纤维环及软骨板），尤其是髓核，有不同程度的退行性改变后，在外力因素或轻微损伤（长期弯腰、负重、下蹲、不良体位等）作用下，椎间盘的纤维环破裂，髓核组织从破裂之处突出（或脱出）于后方或椎管内堆积，导致相邻脊神经根遭受刺激或压迫，从而产生腰部疼痛，伴或不伴有下肢疼痛、麻木、无力，甚至间歇性跛行、大小便功能障碍等一系列症状。椎间盘突出较大，出现椎管狭窄时，患者仅能短距离行走，不能走长路，而且行走时疼痛不能忍受，必须休息片刻后方能再走。

developing symptoms. It's likely that activities such as bending, squatting, lifting heavy objects, coughing forcefully, or prolonged sitting can cause the nucleus pulposus to protrude and compress the nerve, leading to lumbar disc herniation.

Lumbar disc herniation often occurs on the basis of intervertebral disc degeneration. Pathologically, it is mainly due to varying degrees of degenerative changes in various parts of the lumbar intervertebral disc (nucleus pulposus, annulus fibrosus, and cartilage endplate), especially the nucleus pulposus. Under external forces or minor injuries (such as prolonged bending, heavy lifting, squatting, poor posture, etc.), the annulus fibrosus of the intervertebral disc ruptures, and the nucleus pulposus tissue protrudes (or herniates) from the site of rupture posteriorly or into the spinal canal. This leads to stimulation or compression of adjacent spinal nerve roots, resulting in lower back pain, with or without accompanying leg pain, numbness, weakness, and even a series of symptoms such as intermittent claudication and dysfunction of bladder and bowel control. When there is significant disc herniation causing spinal canal narrowing, patients may only be able to walk short distances and cannot tolerate pain while walking, requiring a brief rest before being able to continue.

The vast majority of patients experience disc herniation between L4-L5 and L5-S1 vertebrae. They may simultaneously or individually experience lower back pain and radiating leg pain. Pain exacerbation can be triggered by increased abdominal pressure (such as sneezing, coughing, straining during bowel movements, etc.) or changes in body position, and it may even radiate from the lower back to the legs, manifesting as sciatica. Typical sciatica pain radiates from the lower back to the buttocks, the back of the thigh, the outer side of the lower leg, and down to the foot. In the early stages, symptoms mostly consist of lower back pain, which may lessen after resting for several days or weeks. However, prolonged sitting, labor, or work can cause recurring bouts of lower back pain, which may vary in severity. Mild cases may present with only lower back soreness, discomfort, or fatigue, while severe cases may involve stabbing, burning, or electric shock-like pain that worsens at night. Later-stage symptoms often persist without significant change, and the condition becomes chronic. The protruded disc material becomes fixed by surrounding fibrous tissue, and symptoms may not completely disappear even with rest. Therefore, the location, range, and nature of pain caused by disc herniation can vary depending on factors

绝大多数患者是腰4—5、腰5—骶1间盘突出,腰痛及放射性下肢痛可同时出现,也可单独发生,患者在增加腹压(如打喷嚏、咳嗽、用力排便等)或改变体位时可引发疼痛加重,甚至会从腰部传到下肢,表现为坐骨神经痛。典型坐骨神经痛是从下腰部向臀部、大腿后方、小腿外侧直到足部的放射痛。早期症状多数仅为腰部疼痛,经休息数日或数周后腰痛可减轻,一旦久坐、劳动或工作则腰痛反复发作,时轻时重并有加重趋势,轻者仅有腰部酸痛、胀痛不适或乏力,重者犹如刺痛、灼痛或电击样痛,夜间加重。后期症状多持续不变,病程较长,髓核突出物已被周围纤维组织所固定,即使休息后症状也不能完全消失。因此,腰椎间盘突出症引起疼痛的部位、范围及性质等均可因突出物的大小、部位及病程的长短等因素而不同。一般突出物越大症状越明显。临床上,腰椎间盘突出症常会反复发作,严重困扰我们的工作和生活,因此最好的办法就是预防。

(4)第三腰椎横突综合征。这是临床常见的腰痛原因之一。部分患者告诉医生,自己长期腰痛得厉害,尤其是腰的两边,一按上去就痛得不行,弯腰及旋转腰部时疼痛加剧,疼痛位置固定,误以为是腰肌劳损,多发生在青壮年体力劳动者。第三腰椎横突是腰部肌肉收缩运动的重要支点,此处受力最大,易使肌肉筋脉附着处发生损伤,触诊时,会发现第三腰椎旁边有个条索状硬结。腰部及臀部疼痛常在弯腰、晨起活动时或活动后加重,有时翻身、走路困难,严重的会影响邻近的神经纤维,疼痛向大腿后侧乃至腘窝处扩散,引起下肢放射痛,一般不过膝。常见的病因是急性损伤或慢性劳损,比如,当进行腰椎前屈、侧弯及旋转等动作时,可能导致

such as the size and location of the protrusion and the duration of the condition. Generally, the larger the protrusion, the more prominent the symptoms. Clinically, disc herniation often recurs, significantly affecting work and daily life, so prevention is key.

(4) The third lumbar transverse process syndrome. One of the common causes of lower back pain in clinical practice is the third lumbar transverse process syndrome. Some patients report to the doctor that they have been experiencing severe and localized lower back pain, especially on both sides of the lower back, which intensifies upon bending or rotating the waist. They often mistake it for lumbar muscle strain, and this condition is more prevalent among young adults engaged in physical labor. The third lumbar transverse process is a crucial pivot point for the contraction of the lower back muscles, experiencing the greatest force, which makes it prone to muscle and tendon injuries. Upon palpation, a hard, cord-like structure can be felt next to the third lumbar vertebra. Pain in the lower back and buttocks often worsens in bending, morning activities, or after physical exertion, sometimes causing difficulty in turning over or walking. Severe cases can affect nearby nerve fibers, causing radiating pain to the back of the thigh and even to the popliteal fossa, typically not extending beyond the

knee. Common causes include acute injury or chronic strain. For instance, movements such as forward bending, side bending, and rotation of the lumbar spine may lead to pathological changes in the soft tissues attached to the tip of the transverse process, such as muscle tears and ruptured small blood vessels, resulting in local tissue inflammation, congestion, and exudation. This can further lead to adhesion of surrounding tissues, thickening of fascia, fibrocartilage hyperplasia, compression, and stimulation of the lateral branches of the lumbar nerve, leading to a series of clinical symptoms.

(5) Lumbar spinal stenosis. This is a common condition in the lumbar region that is easily overlooked, more prevalent in middle-aged and elderly individuals, and commonly seen in laborers. However, clinically, there is a trend of lumbar spinal stenosis becoming more common among younger individuals, with secondary causes being predominant, primarily due to degenerative changes in the spine. Apart from age, factors such as bending and lifting, prolonged sitting, high-load work on the lumbar region, and incorrect sitting posture can lead to osteophyte formation in the lumbar vertebrae, intervertebral disc instability, hypertrophy of the ligamentum flavum and vertebral plate, as well as uneven stress on the intervertebral discs,

横突尖端附着的软组织出现病理变化，如肌肉撕裂、小血管破裂等，使局部组织发生炎性肿胀、充血、渗出，进而引起横突周围组织粘连、筋膜增厚、纤维软骨增生，压迫和刺激腰神经后支的外侧支，出现一系列临床症状。

（5）腰椎管狭窄症。这是一种很容易被我们忽视的腰部常见病，多发于中老年人，体力劳动者多见。但是临床上碰到腰椎管狭窄症逐渐年轻化，二三十岁的年轻人逐渐增多，以继发性的病因为主，其中脊柱退行性变是主要发病原因。除了年龄因素外，弯腰负重、久坐和腰部高负荷的工作会导致腰椎骨质增生、椎体间失稳、黄韧带及椎板肥厚，以及不正确的坐姿也可使腰椎间盘的受力不均，压力反复刺激，导致腰椎间盘突出，均可使腰椎管内径缩小，椎管容积变小，达到一定程度后可引起脊神经根或马尾神经受压，导致腰椎管狭窄症，以至于出现间歇性跛行为主要特征的持续性下腰和腿痛和进行性加重的行走活动困难，严重者会出现马尾神经受压损伤的表现。患者在站立、挺腰和行走时，跛行逐渐加重，甚至不能继续行走，坐下或下蹲休息后可缓解，不影响骑自行车。一般情况下，可以通过药物疗法、物理疗法、腰部推拿及练功锻炼缓解症状、增强腰部肌力，有助于腰椎的稳定和防止可能出现的肌肉萎缩。当出现尿频尿急或排尿困难、马鞍区麻木等马尾神经受压症状时，应尽早手术治疗。

（6）产后腰痛。很多年轻妈妈认为生孩子会容易腰痛，所以选择剖宫产，

resulting in repeated pressure and protrusion of the intervertebral discs. These factors can narrow the diameter of the spinal canal and reduce its volume, leading to lumbar spinal stenosis. When it reaches a certain degree, it can cause compression of the spinal nerve roots or the cauda equina nerves, leading to lumbar spinal stenosis. The main characteristics are intermittent claudication, persistent lower back and leg pain aggravated by walking activities, and progressive difficulty in walking. Severe cases may present symptoms of cauda equina nerve compression injury. Patients experience worsening claudication when standing, straightening the back, or walking, and may even become unable to continue walking. Resting by sitting down or squatting can relieve symptoms without affecting cycling. Generally, symptoms can be alleviated and lumbar muscle strength can be enhanced through medication, physical therapy, lumbar massage, and exercise, which helps stabilize the lumbar spine and prevent possible muscle atrophy. However, early surgical treatment is necessary when symptoms of cauda equina nerve compression, such as urinary frequency, urgency, or difficulty, and numbness in the saddle area occur.

(6) Postpartum lower back pain. Many young mothers believe that giving birth will lead to lower back pain, so they opt for

cesarean sections. However, even after a cesarean section, they still experience lower back pain beyond their expectation. In fact, postpartum lower back pain is not directly related to whether the delivery was vaginal or via a cesarean section. During pregnancy, the increase in pregnancy-related hormones causes the ligaments around the pelvis to loosen, increasing the mobility of the lumbosacral joints to facilitate childbirth. However, this also weakens the supporting strength of the lower back, making it susceptible to lower back pain. Additionally, as the fetus and uterus grow during pregnancy, there is increased pressure on the lumbar spine and pelvic floor, affecting the physiological curvature of the lumbar spine and the position of the lumbosacral joints. This pressure can also cause abdominal muscles to stretch, partly leading to abdominal muscle separation, further increasing the burden on the lower back and causing lower back pain. Moreover, postpartum activities such as breastfeeding, carrying the baby, and changing diapers involve prolonged sitting and bending movements, coupled with a lack of exercise, leading to weakening of the back muscles and pelvic floor muscles, which can result in lower back pain.

2. Prevention and Treatment Plan

(1) Changing Unhealthy Habits in Daily Life. Avoid prolonged sitting or

但是剖宫产后还是会出现腰痛，这是让她们没想到的。其实，产后腰痛跟顺产还是剖宫产没有直接联系。在怀孕期间，妊娠相关激素的增加会导致骨盆周围韧带变得松弛，使腰骶部关节活动度增加，有利于孩子的出生，但会使得腰部支撑力量减弱，容易引起腰痛。同时，在怀孕期间，胎儿及子宫逐渐增大，腰腹部负重增加，压迫腰椎和盆底，影响腰椎生理曲度及腰骶部关节位置，以及使得腹肌伸展，部分会出现腹肌分离，进一步导致腰部的负担增加，引起腰痛。另外，产后需要哺乳、抱婴儿、换尿布等久坐、弯腰动作，又缺乏运动锻炼，腰肌及盆底肌肌力减弱，导致腰肌劳损，容易发生腰痛。

2. 防治方案

（1）改变生活中的不良习惯。避免久坐久站，保持良好的坐姿，经常变换体位。注意腰部防寒保暖，避免弯腰负重，床垫软硬适中。加强腰背肌的锻炼，促进气血循环，增强腰部肌肉、韧带弹性。

（2）六字诀功法套路动作。练习整个套路动作，或者侧重反复练习第一式"嘘"字诀，第三式"呼"字诀，第五式"吹"字诀，每个字诀重复练习六遍，每天2次。

3. 习练秘诀

全身放松、精神集中、呼吸平稳，动作要松柔舒缓，配合呼吸、吐音协调自然地去练套路动作，注意每式动作的阴阳转换，促使身体肌肉关节的膨胀然后放松自然地转换。呼吸要求做到"匀、细、柔、长"，吸气时经鼻，每次吸气后不要忙于呼出，宜稍屏片刻，再徐徐呼出。

4. 注意事项

在开始锻炼时，要掌握正确的发音方式；控

standing and maintain a good sitting posture by regularly changing positions. Pay attention to keeping the lower back warm and avoid bending and lifting heavy objects. Ensure that the mattress is of medium firmness. Strengthen the muscles of the lower back to promote blood circulation and enhance the elasticity of the lower back muscles and ligaments.

(2) Liuzijue Routine Movements. Practise the entire routine of exercises, or focus on repeating the first posture "Xu", the third posture "Hu", and the fifth posture "Chui". Practice each posture six times, twice a day.

3. The Secret to Practice

Relax the whole body, focus the mind, and maintain steady breathing. Movements should be gentle and coordinated with breathing, ensuring natural coordination of inhalation and exhalation. Pay attention to the transition of Yin and Yang in each posture, promoting the expansion and natural relaxation of muscles and joints. Breathing should be "even, fine, gentle, and long", inhaling through the nose and not rushing to exhale after each inhalation. It is advisable to pause briefly and then exhale slowly.

4. Points to Note

When starting the exercise, it's important to master correct pronunciation and control the volume, using the level audible to your own ears as a guide. Additionally, adopt abdominal breathing and pursed-lip breathing. Each movement should be gentle and relaxed, gradually increasing the number of repetitions slowly, and avoiding overly prolonged duration. Moreover, the total exercise volume should be adjusted gradually according to individual condition. It's normal to experience slight soreness in the shoulders, waist, and knees in the course of practice.

音量，以自己耳朵能听见的音量为度；采用腹式呼吸、缩唇呼吸；每个动作要松柔舒缓；缓慢地增加运动次数，时间不宜过长。此外，锻炼总量要根据自身情况，逐渐进行增减。在锻炼的过程中会出现肩部、腰部、膝部微微酸痛，这属于正常情况。

第八节 肾　　虚
Section 8　Kidney Deficiency

1. Medical Theories Explained

Kidney deficiency is a collective term for deficiencies in kidney Yang, kidney Yin, kidney Qi, and insufficient kidney Essence. The most common types are kidney Yang deficiency and kidney Yin deficiency, each with distinct clinical manifestations. Kidney Yang deficiency presents with "cold syndrome" symptoms, with aversion to cold being a typical feature. It may also include lower back and knee pain, fatigue, mental fatigue, frequent nocturnal urination, decreased sexual function, erectile

1. 医说析疑

肾虚是肾阳虚、肾阴虚、肾气虚、肾精不足的统称，最常见的有肾阳虚与肾阴虚之分，不同证型的临床表现各有特点。肾阳虚会有"寒证"表现，畏寒怕冷是肾阳虚的一个非常典型的特征，且有腰膝酸冷、神疲体乏、精神萎靡，也会有夜尿频多、性功能减退、男性阳痿、女子月经不调等。肾阴虚的人不会怕冷，但是会有"热证"表现，如腰膝酸软、关节疼痛、手足心发热、盗汗，也会让人变得烦躁不安、脾气暴躁、注意力难以集中、记忆力下降，且常常伴随着失眠、多梦等症。肾虚的原因多与先天不足、脾胃损伤、劳累过度、久病、年老体衰等有关。肾为先天之本，先天之精不足，导致精亏、肾虚。因为脾为后天之本，可以营养五脏六腑，充养先天之精，现在的上班族经常饮食不节，长期食用高盐高糖、重油重辣、冰凉刺激的食物和饮料，容易损伤脾胃功能，久而久之就伤及肾脏。另外，劳累过度、情志失调的影响，例如，工作长期处于高负荷的状态，让大脑得不到休息，就易损耗"髓海"，髓海空虚，脑失所养，久之影响肾精不足；另有，纵欲过度，房事过多，容易导致阳气耗损过多、肾精流失，最终引发肾亏。还有老年人由于年老体衰，肾精及肾气逐渐衰减，最终引发肾虚。在人体病理过程中，也会影响累及肾

dysfunction in men, and irregular menstruation in women. In contrast, individuals with kidney Yin deficiency do not fear cold but exhibit "heat syndrome" symptoms, such as lower back and knee weakness, joint pain, hot sensations in the palms and soles, night sweats, irritability, restlessness, difficulty concentrating, memory decline, and often insomnia and vivid dreaming. The causes of kidney deficiency are often related to congenital deficiencies, spleen and stomach damage, excessive fatigue, prolonged illness, and aging. The kidney is the root of congenital essence, and congenital essence deficiency leads to essence depletion and kidney deficiency. The spleen is the root of acquired essence and can nourish the congenital essence. Nowadays, many office workers have irregular diets, consuming high-salt, high-sugar, greasy, and spicy foods and beverages, which can easily damage the spleen and stomach function, ultimately affecting the kidneys. Additionally, excessive fatigue and emotional imbalance, such as prolonged high-stress work, can deplete the "marrow sea," leading to insufficient nourishment of the brain and eventually affecting kidney essence. Furthermore, excessive indulgence and frequent sexual activity can deplete Yang Qi and kidney essence, eventually leading to kidney deficiency. For the elderly, due to old age and physical decline, kidney essense and kidney Qi gradually decline, and finally lead to kidney deficiency. Moreover, in the pathological process of the human body, prolonged illness can affect the Essence, Qi, Yin, and Yang of the kidneys, making it one of the causes of kidney deficiency. Some studies suggest that immune function is reduced in a state of kidney deficiency.

2. Prevention and Treatment Plan

(1) Changing Unhealthy Habits in Daily Life. Pay attention to moderate sexual activity and keep the lower back and abdomen warm. Maintain a calm mindset, avoid negative emotions such as worry, anxiety, and fear, as they can harm the body. Maintain regular daily routines and learn to adjust them accordingly. Practice moderation in diet, avoid overeating, and avoid critical addiction to certain foods.

(2) Liuzijue Routine Movements. Practise the entire routine of exercises, or focus on repeating the fifth posture "Chui". Practice the posture six times, twice a day.

3. The Secret to Practice

Relax the whole body, concentrate the mind, and maintain steady breathing. Perform movements gently and smoothly, coordinating with breath and sound, ensuring a natural flow. Pay attention to the transition between Yin and Yang in each posture, promoting the expansion and relaxation of

之精气阴阳，故久病伤肾也是肾虚原因之一。有研究认为，在肾虚的状态下，肾脏的免疫力降低。

2. 防治方案

（1）改变生活中的不良习惯。注意性生活适度，腰腹部要注意保暖。要注意心态平和，避免忧愁、思虑、惊恐等不良情绪。作息规律，懂得调节。饮食要有节制，不能暴饮暴食，不能对食物过分偏嗜。

（2）六字诀功法套路动作。练习整个套路动作，或者侧重反复练习第五式"吹"字诀，此字诀重复练习六遍，每天2次。

3. 习练秘诀

全身放松、精神集中、呼吸平稳，动作要松柔舒缓，配合呼吸、吐音协调自然地去练套路动作，注意每式动作的阴阳转换，促使身体肌肉关节的膨胀然后放松自然地转换。呼吸要求做到"匀、细、柔、长",吸气时经鼻,每次吸气后不要忙于呼出,宜稍屏片刻,再徐徐呼出。按五行相生次序排列,"吹"与肾相对应,肾主冬,冬季可以多锻炼"吹"字功,具有调理肾脏功能的作用,可以滋养肾脏及改善阳虚性慢性疾病,如肺病、心脏病、胃肠病、骨关节病等。运用腹式呼吸,会使气息流畅,产生柔和的内脏按摩作用,从而改善肾脏功能。

4. 注意事项

在开始锻炼时,要掌握正确的发音方式;控制音量,以自己耳朵能听见的音量为度;采用腹式呼吸、缩唇呼吸;每个动作要松柔舒缓;缓慢地增加运动次数,时间不宜过长。此外,锻炼总量要根据自身情况,逐渐进行增减。在锻炼的过程中会出现肩部、膝部微微酸痛,这属于正常情况。

muscles and joints naturally. Breathe evenly, gently, softly, and deeply, inhaling through the nose. After each inhalation, avoid immediate exhalation, pause briefly, then exhale slowly. Following the sequence of the Five Elements, "Chui" corresponds to the kidneys. The kidneys govern winter, so practicing the "Chui" posture more in winter can regulate kidney function, nourish the kidneys, and improve chronic conditions related to Yang deficiency, such as respiratory, cardiovascular, gastrointestinal, and musculoskeletal disorders. Employing abdominal breathing facilitates smooth airflow and gentle internal organs massage, enhancing visceral function.

4. Points to Note

When starting the exercise, it's important to master correct pronunciation and control the volume, using the level audible to your own ears as a guide. Employ abdominal breathing and pursed-lip breathing. Each movement should be gentle, relaxed, and slow, gradually increasing the number of repetitions, and avoiding excessively long durations. Additionally, the overall exercise intensity should be adjusted according to individual condition, gradually increasing or decreasing as needed. It's normal to experience slight soreness in the shoulders and knees in the course of practice.

第九节　胃肠功能紊乱
Section 9　Gastrointestinal Dysfunction

1. Medical Theories Explained

Gastrointestinal functional disorders are very common in our daily lives. Patients often describe symptoms such as feeling hungry but getting full quickly after eating a little, loss of appetite for favorite foods, alternating diarrhea and constipation, feeling the urge to defecate but unable to, frequent bloating, belching, lack of appetite, upper abdominal burning sensation, and nausea. Despite undergoing various examinations at hospitals and being told that everything is normal. In fact, the appearance of these discomfort symptoms often indicates a disturbance in gastrointestinal function. This condition is the most common functional gastrointestinal disorder. In traditional Chinese medicine, it can be categorized into various patterns, such as liver Qi stagnation, liver Qi invading the stomach, spleen-stomach Qi deficiency, damp-heat stagnating in the stomach, and mixed cold and heat patterns. It is also easily influenced by seasonal changes. For example, during the spring season with frequent climate fluctuations and unstable temperatures, the body is susceptible to external stimuli,

1. 医说析疑

胃肠功能紊乱在我们的生活中很常见，患者的不适症状常常描述有明明肚子很饿，却吃一点就饱了；平时爱吃的菜，这几天却对它没胃口；前段时间拉稀，最近又便秘；总感觉有大便，到厕所却拉不出；时常饱胀、嗳气、食欲缺乏、上腹灼热、犯恶心。以上种种不适，去医院做各种检查又提示正常，其实这类不适症状的出现，往往提示胃肠功能已经紊乱。该病为胃肠道最常见的功能性胃肠病，中医辨证可分为肝气郁结证、肝气犯胃证、脾胃气虚证、湿热滞胃证、寒热错杂证等证型。也易受季节更替影响，如春季气候变化频繁、温度不稳定，人体易受外界刺激而引发腹泻、肠炎等肠胃疾病。平素可以多吃一些温热好消化的食物。

leading to conditions like diarrhea and enteritis. It is advisable to consume more warm and easily digestible foods in daily life.

2. 防治方案

（1）改变生活中的不良习惯。生活有规律，按时作息，起居有常，避免熬夜，不妄劳作，保证充足的睡眠。每天坚持运动锻炼，保持心情舒畅。调整饮食结构，饮食宜定时、适量，建议低脂肪及少食多餐，避免刺激性食物。

（2）六字诀功法套路动作。反复练习整个套路动作，或侧重练习第一式"嘘"字诀，第三式"呼"字诀，第六式"嘻"字诀，每个字诀重复练习六遍，每天2次。

3. 习练秘诀

全身放松、精神集中、呼吸平稳，动作要松柔舒缓，配合呼吸、吐音协调自然地去练套路动作，注意每式动作的阴阳转换，促使身体肌肉关节的膨胀然后放松自然地转换。呼吸要求做到"匀、细、柔、长"，吸气时经鼻，每次吸气后不要忙于呼出，宜

2. Prevention and Treatment Plan

(1) Changing Unhealthy Habits in Daily Life. Maintain a regular lifestyle, adhering to a consistent schedule and avoiding staying up late. Ensure adequate sleep and avoid overexertion. Engage in daily exercise and keep a cheerful mood. Adjust your diet by eating at regular intervals and in appropriate amounts. It is recommended to consume low-fat foods and have smaller, more frequent meals. Avoid stimulating foods.

(2) Liuzijue Routine Movements. Practise the entire routine of exercises, or focus on practicing the first posture "Xu", the third posture "Hu", and the sixth posture "Xi". Practice each posture six times, twice a day.

3. The Secret to Practice

Relax your whole body, focus your mind, and maintain steady breathing. Perform the movements smoothly and gently, coordinating them naturally with your breathing and vocalization. Pay attention to the Yin-Yang transitions in each posture to promote the expansion and relaxation of your muscles and joints. Your breathing should be even, fine, gentle, and long. Inhale through your nose, hold your breath for a moment after each inhalation, then exhale slowly. Spring is a peak season for triggering gastrointestinal discomfort such as bloating, loss of appetite, abdominal pain, diarrhea, constipation, and enteritis, which can contribute to gastrointestinal disorders. Following the sequence of Five Elements, "Xu" corresponds to the Liver, which is associated with Wood and spring. Practicing the "Xu" sound exercise can help regulate the Liver meridian and improve liver function, thereby alleviating symptoms of Liver Qi stagnation and Liver Qi attacking the stomach. Employing abdominal breathing facilitates smooth airflow and gentle internal organs massage, enhancing visceral function.

4. Points to Note

When starting to practice, it is important to master the correct pronunciation and control the volume, ensuring it is audible to your own ears. Use abdominal breathing and pursed-lip breathing techniques. Each movement should be performed smoothly and gently, and the number of repetitions should be increased gradually, ensuring the duration is not too long at the beginning. Additionally, the total amount of exercise should be adjusted according to your own condition, increasing or decreasing gradually. It's normal to experience slight soreness in the shoulders and knees in the course of practice.

稍屏片刻，再徐徐呼出。春季是易诱发饱胀不适、食欲不振、腹痛、腹泻、便秘、肠炎等肠胃疾病的高发季节，这也增加了肠胃紊乱的可能性。按五行相生次序排列，"嘘"与肝相对应，肝属木，相应于春，锻炼"嘘"字功，具有疏通肝经、调理肝脏功能的作用，可以改善肝气郁结证、肝气犯胃证之痞满。运用腹式呼吸，会使气息流畅，产生柔和的内脏按摩作用，从而改善内脏功能。

4. 注意事项

在开始锻炼时，要掌握正确的发音方式；控制音量，以自己耳朵能听见的音量为度；采用腹式呼吸、缩唇呼吸；每个动作要松柔舒缓；缓慢地增加运动次数，时间不宜过长。此外，锻炼总量要根据自身情况，逐渐进行增减。在锻炼的过程中会出现肩部、膝部微微酸痛，这属于正常情况。

第十节 骨质疏松症
Section 10　Osteoporosis

1. 医说析疑

骨质疏松症是老年人中最常见的骨骼疾病，一种以骨量低、骨微结构损坏，导致骨骼脆性增加、易发生骨折为特征的全身性骨病。这是一种与增龄相关的骨骼疾病，随着人口老龄化，老年骨质疏松症发病率日益增高，常常导致疼痛、驼背或身高变矮等脊柱变形，其最严重后果就是骨质疏松性骨折。但是老年人对骨质疏松症认知普遍不足，他们经常因为腰背部疼痛来就医，误以为是劳累、搬重物或扭伤引起的疼痛，但是弯腰、翻身时疼痛加剧，痛得起不了床，上床也困难，行动受限，卧床休息时疼痛可以减轻，但是变换体位时疼痛又明显加重了，无法继续日常生活和工作。这是一种难以察觉的疾病，因为发作前没有明显的迹象或症状，直到骨折时引

1. Medical Theories Explained

Osteoporosis is the most common skeletal disease among the elderly. It is characterized by low bone mass and the deterioration of bone microarchitecture, leading to increased bone fragility and a higher risk of fractures. This age-related skeletal condition is becoming increasingly prevalent as the population ages. Osteoporosis in the elderly often results in pain, kyphosis, or reduced height due to spinal deformities, with osteoporotic fractures being the most severe consequence. However, awareness of osteoporosis among the elderly is generally low. Elderly patients often seek medical help for back pain, mistakenly attributing it to fatigue, heavy lifting, or sprains. Yet, the pain worsens when bending over or turning in bed, to the point where getting out of bed is difficult, and daily activities are severely limited. Pain may subside with bed rest but intensifies significantly with movement, hindering daily life and work. Osteoporotic fractures are often overlooked as a cause of such pain because the disease is insidious, with no apparent signs or symptoms until a fracture occurs and causes severe pain. In elderly individuals, even minor falls, slight impacts, sudden movements, or actions such as coughing, bending over, or lifting objects can lead to fractures due to osteoporosis.

In outpatient clinics, the doctor often encounters patients who say they drink milk and take calcium supplements daily, yet still develop osteoporosis. This misunderstanding stems from the belief that calcium supplementation alone is sufficient. The fundamental preventive measures include maintaining a healthy lifestyle, engaging in appropriate exercise, and preventing falls. Additionally, it is essential to choose suitable types of exercise, intensity, and duration based on individual conditions, and to progress gradually. Moderate exercise can improve bone density and bone quality while also enhancing muscle strength and balance, thereby reducing the risk of falls and fractures. These activities exert additional stress on bones, stimulating bone growth.

2. Prevention and Treatment Plan

(1) Changing Unhealthy Habits in Daily Life. Pay attention to mental health regulation, control weight, and avoid obesity to reduce the burden on the spine. Avoid smoking, excessive alcohol consumption, and coffee. Maintain a balanced diet, consume calcium-rich food, and get plenty

起剧烈疼痛才会被发现。骨质疏松症老年患者生活中碰到的跌倒、轻微撞击、突发性的动作,甚至咳嗽、弯腰或抬举物件都有可能造成骨折。

门诊中也经常碰到患者说自己天天喝牛奶和补钙片了,怎么还会骨质疏松呢?这是他们认识不足,误以为单单补钙就够了。基础预防措施是健康的生活方式、适当运动、预防跌倒。除此之外,根据个人情况选择合适的锻炼方式、锻炼强度和时间,循序渐进,适当运动可以提高骨密度和骨质量,同时增加肌肉力量及平衡能力,降低发生跌倒及骨折的风险。这些运动可以给骨骼带来额外负荷,刺激骨骼生长。

2. 防治方案

(1)改变生活中的不良习惯。注重心理健康调节,控制体重,避免肥胖,减轻脊柱负重,避免吸烟、过度饮酒、咖啡,均衡营养,多吃含钙的食物,多晒太阳,避免久坐、久卧、弯腰、负重、受寒，适当的体育活动，增强腰背肌。

（2）六字诀功法套路动作。反复练习整个套路动作，每个字诀重复练习六遍，每天2次。

3. 习练秘诀

全身放松、精神集中、呼吸平稳，动作要松柔舒缓，配合呼吸、吐音协调自然地去练套路动作，注意每式动作的阴阳转换，促使身体肌肉关节的膨胀然后放松自然地转换。呼吸要求做到"匀、细、柔、长"，吸气时经鼻，每次吸气后不要忙于呼出，宜稍屏片刻，再徐徐呼出。春季多锻炼"嘘"字功，按五行相生次序排列，"嘘"与肝相对应，肝属木，相应于春，锻炼"嘘"字功，具有疏通肝经、调理肝脏功能的作用，可以改善肝气郁结证，使心情愉快。运用腹式呼吸，会使气息流畅，产生柔和的内脏按摩作用，从而改善内脏功能。

of sunlight. Avoid prolonged sitting, lying down, bending over, heavy lifting, and exposure to cold. Engage in appropriate physical activities to strengthen the muscles of the lower back.

(2) Liuzijue Routine Movements. Practice the entire routine of exercises, repeating each posture six times, twice a day.

3. The Secret to Practice

Relax your whole body, focus your mind, and maintain steady breathing. Perform the movements smoothly and gently, coordinating them naturally with your breathing and sound production. Pay attention to the Yin-Yang transitions in each movement, allowing your muscles and joints to expand and then relax naturally. Breathing requirements should be "even, fine, gentle, and long". Inhale through the nose, hold your breath briefly after each inhalation, and then exhale slowly. In spring, practice the "Xu" posture more frequently. Following the sequence of Five Elements, "Xu" corresponds to the Liver, which belongs to Wood and is associated with spring. Practicing the "Xu" sound helps to regulate the Liver meridian and improve Liver function, which can improve Liver Qi stagnation and promote a happy mood. Employing abdominal breathing facilitates smooth airflow and gentle internal organs massage, enhancing visceral function.

4. Points to Note

When beginning your practice, it is important to master the correct pronunciation and control the volume, ensuring it is audible to your own ears. Use abdominal breathing and pursed-lip breathing techniques. Each movement should be smooth and gentle, and the number of repetitions should be increased slowly. The duration of each session should not last too long initially. Additionally, the total amount of exercise should be adjusted according to your own condition, gradually increasing or decreasing as needed. It is normal to experience mild soreness in the shoulders and knees in the course of practice.

4. 注意事项

在开始锻炼时，要掌握正确的发音方式；控制音量，以自己耳朵能听见的音量为度；采用腹式呼吸、缩唇呼吸；每个动作要松柔舒缓；缓慢地增加运动次数，时间不宜过长。此外，锻炼总量要根据自身情况，逐渐进行增减。在锻炼的过程中会出现肩部、膝部微微酸痛，这属于正常情况。

第十一节 脂 肪 肝
Section 11 Fatty Liver

1. Medical Theories Explained

Fatty liver refers to the diffuse fat infiltration of liver cells caused by excessive accumulation of fat in the body or long-term heavy alcohol drinking. Different types of fatty liver present with different clinical manifestations. The most common fatty

1. 医说析疑

脂肪肝是指由于体内脂肪堆积过多或长期大量饮酒等多种原因引起的肝细胞弥漫性脂肪变。不同类型的脂肪肝，具有不同的临床表现。脂肪肝临床上最常见的就是非酒精性脂肪性肝病，这类患者大多体型肥胖，一般都是由于大量摄入高油、高脂、高盐、高糖的食物以及久坐、缺乏运动锻炼等不健康的生活方式所至。另外，很多又瘦又年轻的患者怎么也想不明白自己怎么就得了脂肪肝。大家发现自己患有脂肪肝的过程，一般都是在某次常规体检报告中突然出现了脂肪肝。刚查出来的时候，心里可能会紧张一下，可这个病本人没啥感觉，大部分人低估这个疾病，时间一长甚至都给忘了。早期的脂肪肝病变是可逆转的，所以一定要及时干预，可以去看专科医生做进一步检查，比如，肝硬化指数、肝功血液指标、肝脏组织活检之类的方法，可以筛查和排除肝纤维化乃至肝硬化。

脂肪肝如果不加以控制，可逐渐进展为脂肪性肝炎、肝硬化，甚至肝癌。根据肝细胞脂肪变程度，脂肪肝可分为轻度、中度、重度三种类型。轻度脂肪肝大多无临床症状，肝功

liver in clinical practice is non-alcoholic fatty liver disease. Most patients with this condition are obese, often due to unhealthy dietary habits characterized by high oil, high fat, high salt, and high sugar intake, as well as sedentary lifestyles and lack of exercise. Additionally, many thin and young patients cannot understand why they have fatty liver. The process of discovering one's fatty liver condition typically occurs when a fatty liver is unexpectedly identified in an abdominal ultrasound report during a routine physical examination. When first diagnosed, individuals may feel a moment of anxiety, but since they often do not experience any symptoms, many people underestimate the seriousness of this disease, and over time, they may even forget about it. Early-stage fatty liver disease is reversible, so timely intervention is essential. Patients can seek further examinations by visiting a specialist, such as liver fibrosis index tests, liver function tests, liver tissue biopsies, and other methods to screen for and exclude liver fibrosis or even cirrhosis.

If left uncontrolled, fatty liver can gradually progress to non-alcoholic steatohepatitis, cirrhosis, and even liver cancer. Based on the degree of hepatocellular fat infiltration, fatty liver can be classified into three types: mild, moderate, and severe. Mild fatty liver mostly presents with no clinical symptoms, and liver function tests are generally normal, although individuals may experience fatigue and are often obese. Studies have shown that for mild fatty liver, weight reduction can significantly decrease liver fat content in most patients and even alleviate the severity of fatty liver hepatitis. Moderate fatty liver may manifest as discomfort in the liver area, loss of appetite, and mild abnormalities in liver function. Severe fatty liver is characterized by liver or right upper abdominal pain, fatigue, abnormal liver function tests, elevated transaminases, as well as clinical signs such as spider angiomas and jaundice.

2. Prevention and Treatment Plan

(1) Changing Unhealthy Habits in Daily Life. Control weight and waist circumference, exercise more to increase the basal metabolic rate. Adjust your diet, avoid high-fat, high-sugar, and high-carbohydrate diets, maintain a low-sugar, low-fat diet, eat more vegetables and fruits, and increase dietary fiber intake. Avoid alcohol and avoid staying up late.

(2) Liuzijue Routine Movements. Repeatedly practice the entire routine movements, or focus on practicing the first posture "Xu", the third posture "Hu", and the sixth posture "Xi". Repeat each posture six times, twice a day.

能检查基本都是正常的，多有疲乏感，大多体型肥胖。有关研究表明，对于轻度脂肪肝，减轻体重可以使大部分脂肪肝患者的肝脂肪含量明显减少，甚至脂肪型肝炎的程度都能减轻。中度脂肪肝会感觉到肝区不适，食欲不振，肝功能轻度异常等表现。重度脂肪肝有肝区或右上腹疼痛，疲倦乏力，肝功能检查异常、转氨酶升高，还会有蜘蛛痣、黄疸等临床表现。

2. 防治方案

（1）改变生活中的不良习惯。控制体重和腰围，多做运动，增加基础代谢率。饮食调整，避免高脂、高糖和高碳水化合物饮食，保持低糖低脂饮食，多吃蔬菜和水果，增加膳食纤维。戒酒，不要熬夜。

（2）六字诀功法套路动作。反复练习整个套路动作，或侧重练习第一式"嘘"字诀，第三式"呼"字诀，第六式"嘻"字诀，每个字诀重复练习六遍，每天2次。

3. 习练秘诀

全身放松、精神集中、呼吸平稳，动作要松柔舒缓，配合呼吸、吐音协调自然地去练套路动作，注意每式动作的阴阳转换，促使身体肌肉关节的膨胀然后放松自然地转换。呼吸要求做到"匀、细、柔、长"，吸气时经鼻，每次吸气后不要忙于呼出，宜稍屏片刻，再徐徐呼出。按五行相生次序排列，"嘘"与肝相对应，肝属木，相应于春，多锻炼"嘘"字功，具有疏通肝经、调理肝脏功能的作用，可以改善肝气郁结证，使心情愉快。运用腹式呼吸，会使气息流畅，产生柔和的内脏按摩作用，从而改善内脏功能。

4. 注意事项

在开始锻炼时，要掌握正确的发音方式；控制音量，以自己耳朵能听见的音量为度；采用腹式呼吸、缩唇呼吸；每个动作要松柔舒缓；缓慢地增加运动次数，时间不宜过长。此外，锻炼总量要根据自

3. The Secret to Practice

Relax the whole body, concentrate the mind, maintain steady breathing. Perform the movements gently and smoothly, coordinating with the breath and the exhalation of sounds, in a natural and harmonious manner. Pay attention to the transformation of Yin and Yang in each posture, facilitating the natural expansion and relaxation of muscles and joints. The breath should be "even, fine, soft, and long", inhaling through the nose, and after each inhalation, refrain from exhaling immediately. Instead, pause briefly before exhaling slowly. According to the sequence of the Five Elements, "Xu" corresponds to the Liver, which belongs to Wood and is associated with spring. Practicing "Xu" can effectively regulate the Liver meridian, improving Liver Qi stagnation, and fostering a cheerful disposition. Employing abdominal breathing facilitates smooth airflow and gentle internal organs massage, enhancing visceral function.

4. Points to Note

When starting exercise, it's important to master correct pronunciation and control volume, using the level of sound audible to oneself as a guide. Employ abdominal breathing and pursed-lip breathing. Each movement should be gentle and relaxed, gradually increasing the number of repetitions and avoiding excessive duration.

Additionally, adjust the total amount of exercise according to individual condition, gradually increasing or decreasing as needed. It's normal to experience slight soreness in the shoulders and knees in the course of practice.

第十二节　膝　　痛
Section 12　Knee Pain

1. Medical Theories Explained

The knee joint is one of the most complex and important joints in our body. It bears the weight of our body and is involved in daily activities. However, the knee joint is very vulnerable. Once injured, it tends to recur and may even worsen over time, with slow self-recovery. Therefore, knee joint maintenance is particularly important. This condition is common among middle-aged and elderly people. The knee joint, as a crucial joint supporting our walking and running, can suffer from wear and tear due to factors such as exposure to cold, obesity, and improper exercise, leading to knee pain, swelling, and limited range of motion. In daily activities or sports, every movement involves the participation of the knee joint. Therefore, after each movement, more or

以在每一个动作完成后，或多或少会对膝关节的软骨造成损伤。比如，坐得久时（如办公、看书、看电视时），会感觉前膝疼痛，需要偶尔伸直膝关节来舒缓不适。疼痛原因是坐着时，膝盖较贴近股关节沟，增加了膝盖承受的压力，站起身时，前膝疼痛亦会加剧。

膝关节炎是由慢性损伤、肥胖、老化、代谢异常、营养的改变等因素引起的关节炎性病变，主要临床特征是关节红、肿、热、痛和功能障碍。膝关节的早期不适有多种形式，包括轻微的酸痛、肿胀、软弱或弹响声、摩擦音或摩擦感。随着时间的积累及关节退变，症状逐渐变得频繁，膝关节出现肿胀、疼痛、活动幅度减少、下蹲变得困难。在膝关节部位还常患有膝关节骨性关节炎、膝关节滑膜炎、膝关节半月板损伤、膝关节韧带损伤、髌下脂肪垫劳损、股四头肌肌腱炎、髌腱损伤、髌骨软化症、髌周滑囊炎等关节疾病。

（1）膝骨关节炎。这

less damage may be caused to the cartilage of the knee joint. For example, prolonged sitting, such as working, reading, or watching TV, may cause anterior knee pain, requiring occasional knee extension to alleviate discomfort. The reason for the pain is that when one sits, the knee is closer to the femoral groove, increasing the pressure on the knee. When one stands up, the anterior knee pain may worsen.

Knee arthritis is an inflammatory condition of the joint caused by chronic injury, obesity, aging, metabolic abnormalities, and changes in nutrition. The main clinical features include joint redness, swelling, heat, pain, and functional impairment. Early discomfort in the knee can manifest in various forms, including mild soreness, swelling, weakness, or crepitus, as well as friction sounds or sensations. Over time and with joint degeneration, these symptoms become more frequent, leading to swelling, pain, reduced range of motion, and difficulty squatting. In the knee area, several joint diseases are commonly observed, such as osteoarthritis of the knee, synovitis of the knee, meniscal injuries, ligament injuries, infrapatellar fat pad syndrome, quadriceps tendonitis, patellar tendon injuries, chondromalacia patellae, and peripatellar bursitis.

(1) Knee Osteoarthritis. Knee

osteoarthritis is a chronic joint disease characterized by degenerative changes in the knee joint cartilage and secondary bone hypertrophy. It predominantly affects middle-aged and elderly individuals, particularly those over 50 years old, and is more common in women. This condition is a primary cause of leg pain and difficulty in walking among the elderly. Other contributing factors include being overweight, improper walking posture, prolonged squatting, long-term mountain-climbing, stair climbing, exposure to cold and damp conditions, and frequent joint injuries. Additionally, overuse of the joints, such as in heavy manual labor or professional athletes, as well as individuals with joint instability or meniscus injuries, are also prone to developing knee osteoarthritis.

The knee joint not only supports the body's weight but also endures the frequent movements required in daily life, such as walking and running, making it susceptible to wear and tear. Its primary characteristics include subchondral bone thickening, cartilage degradation, and the formation of bone spurs. The main clinical manifestations are joint pain, swelling, limited joint mobility, crepitus, joint deformities, and muscle atrophy. In daily life, many patients with knee osteoarthritis experience severe pain, stiffness, and movement difficulties,

是一种以膝关节软骨退行性变和继发性骨质增生为特征的慢性关节疾病，多发于50岁以上的中老年人，多见于女性。此病是常常困扰老年人腿疼和行走困难的主要原因。另外，体重超标、不正确的走路姿势、长时间下蹲、长期进行登山、上下楼梯、膝关节的受凉受寒以及经常性关节损伤也是导致膝关节炎的原因。还有，关节过度使用，如重体力劳动者、职业运动员等人群，以及存在关节不稳、半月板损伤等关节损伤的人群，也容易发生膝骨关节炎。

膝关节不仅要支撑全身的重量，还需要承担日常生活中频繁进行的动作，例如走路、跑步等，因此很容易发生劳损，其特征主要是软骨下骨增厚，关节软骨退化和骨赘形成。主要临床表现是关节疼痛、肿胀，关节活动受限，骨摩擦音，关节畸形、肌肉萎缩。生活中，不少膝关节炎患者在昼夜温差大，倒春寒来袭时，就会出现疼痛难忍、僵硬不适和运动障碍的症状,并且有久站不舒服、爬楼梯不舒服、一走长路就膝疼、蹲不下去、膝盖一旦变天就疼得厉害等不适,甚至坐久了都觉得膝盖腘窝处胀胀的。

(2)膝关节滑膜炎。目前无论是老年人还是青少年,膝关节滑膜炎的发病率越来越高,是一种常见的炎症性疾病,大部分还是因为退化和磨损引起的无菌性滑膜炎,主要表现为膝关节肿胀、疼痛,还可能会伴有发热、皮肤温度升高、关节活动受限等症状。膝关节滑膜炎有急性与慢性之分。急性滑膜炎,多数是因外伤史引起的急性发作,发病关节周围会出现红肿、灼热、疼痛等症状,且关节活动明显受限,活动时感到疼痛剧烈,伸直或大幅度弯曲时尤甚,检查时压痛点不定。慢性滑膜炎,一般有外伤史,还有本身关节的退行性变和长期久坐久站、下蹲引起的关节磨损,

especially during significant temperature fluctuations or sudden cold snaps in early spring. Symptoms often include discomfort after prolonged standing, difficulty climbing stairs, knee pain after walking long distances, inability to squat, and increased pain during weather changes. Even sitting for extended periods can cause a feeling of tightness in the popliteal area behind the knee.

(2) Knee Synovitis. Currently, the incidence of knee synovitis is increasing among both the elderly and young people. This common inflammatory disease is mostly caused by degeneration and wear, leading to aseptic synovitis. Its primary symptoms include knee joint swelling and pain, which may be accompanied by fever, increased skin temperature, and restricted joint movement. Knee synovitis can be classified into acute and chronic types. Acute synovitis is mostly triggered by a history of trauma, resulting in acute onset. The affected joint area shows symptoms such as redness, swelling, heat, and pain, with a significant limitation in joint movement. Patients experience severe pain when excercising, especially when extending or bending the knee extensively. The tenderness points are often not fixed for the check. Chronic synovitis generally arises from a history of trauma, coupled with joint degeneration and long periods of sitting or

standing, as well as squatting, which cause joint wear. Symptoms include joint swelling and pain, though these are less severe than in acute synovitis. Patients may have difficulty performing squatting movements, and symptoms often worsen after fatigue but improve with rest. The skin temperature is usually normal. As the disease progresses, the synovial sac wall may thicken, leading to joint instability and affecting normal joint function, which restricts regular activities. For acute synovitis, immobilization and adequate rest are crucial treatments to reduce the secretion of synovial fluid and promote its absorption. Additionally, strengthening exercises for the quadriceps (thigh muscles) are essential to prevent muscle atrophy.

(3) Knee Meniscus Injury. This is a common type of injury in sports. It is frequently observed in young and middle-aged adults, mainly in male patients. After meniscus injury, symptoms such as pain, swelling, popping, and locking often occur. For instance, varying degrees of knee pain, painful popping while walking, a tendency for the knee to suddenly "lock" when bending or straightening, increased pain when climbing stairs, squatting, running, or jumping, and sudden weakness in the knee leading to a "giving a way" sensation may be experienced. Most patients have a history of twisting injury, such as playing

关节周围也会出现肿胀、疼痛，程度稍轻，做下蹲动作有困难，往往劳累后会加重，休息过后症状会减轻，皮肤温度多为正常。随着病程的发展，滑膜囊壁会出现增厚现象，关节不稳固，影响关节的正常功能，导致正常活动受到限制。制动、充分休息，是滑膜炎急性发作的重要治疗方式，这样可以使滑膜液体的分泌减少，同时促进滑液的吸收，除此之外，还要加强股四头肌（大腿肌肉）的锻炼，防止肌肉萎缩。

（3）膝关节半月板损伤。这是运动损伤中常见的一种损伤。临床上多见于青壮年，主要是男性患者，半月板损伤后常出现疼痛、肿胀、弹响、交锁等症状，比如膝关节不同程度疼痛，走路时常有痛性弹响，膝关节弯曲到伸直或伸直到弯曲时容易发生突然"卡住"的现象，上下楼、下蹲、跑、跳时疼痛更明显，也有可能突发膝关节无力，出现"打软腿"现象。大部分患者膝关节都会有扭伤史,比如打篮球、踢足球、跆拳道、武术等。半月板是一个纤维软骨,具有吸收震荡、缓冲压力、润滑和稳定膝关节,避免关节软骨发生磨损的作用。但是半月板抗压不抗旋,容易受扭转外力而出现破裂,破坏结构完整性,导致关节失稳。半月板血液供应非常差,仅有外侧1/3区域来自关节囊的血供,所以损伤后的半月板很难恢复至正常。

2. 防治方案

(1) 改变生活中的不良习惯。注意膝关节防寒保暖。避免长时间站立、步行、下蹲,避免剧烈运动,避免过多爬山、爬楼梯等活动。控制体重、避免辛辣刺激性食物、均衡营养饮食。

(2) 六字诀功法套路动作。反复练习整个套路动作,每个字诀重复练习六遍,每天2次。

3. 习练秘诀

全身放松、精神集中、呼吸平稳,动作要松柔舒缓,配合呼吸、吐音协调

basketball, soccer, taekwondo, martial arts, and so forth. The meniscus is a fibrous cartilage structure that absorbs shock, cushions pressure, lubricates, and stabilizes the knee joint, preventing wear and tear of the articular cartilage. However, the meniscus is susceptible to torsional forces and can easily tear under such external forces, disrupting its structural integrity and causing joint instability. Blood supply to the meniscus is very poor, with only about one-third of the outer region receiving blood from the joint capsule. Therefore, recovery to normalcy after a meniscus injury is usually difficult.

2. Prevention and Treatment Plan

(1) Changing Unhealthy Habits in Daily Life. Keep knee joint warmth and protection against cold. Avoid prolonged standing, walking, and squatting, as well as intense physical activities and excessive climbing of hills or stairs. Maintain a healthy body weight and refrain from consuming spicy or stimulating food, opting instead for a balanced and nutritious diet.

(2) Liuzijue Routine Movements. Repeatedly practice the entire routine, each posture six times, twice a day.

3. The Secret to Practice

Relax the whole body, concentrate the mind, maintain steady breathing. Perform the movements gently and smoothly, coordinating with the breath and the sound of exhalation naturally. Pay attention to the transformation of Yin and Yang in each posture, promoting the expansion and relaxation of muscles and joints. The breathing should be "even, fine, gentle, and long", inhaling through the nose. After each inhalation, do not rush to exhale, instead, pause briefly and then exhale slowly.

4. Points to Note

When starting the exercise, it's important to master correct pronunciation and control the volume, using the level that you can hear with your own ears as a guide. Adopt abdominal breathing and pursed-lip breathing. Each movement should be gentle and relaxed, gradually increasing the number of repetitions slowly, and avoiding excessively long durations. Additionally, the total amount of exercise should be adjusted gradually based on individual condition. It's normal to experience slight soreness in the knees in the course of practice.

自然地去练套路动作，注意每式动作的阴阳转换，促使身体肌肉关节的膨胀然后放松自然地转换。呼吸要求做到"匀、细、柔、长"，吸气时经鼻，每次吸气后不要忙于呼出，宜稍屏片刻，再徐徐呼出。

4. 注意事项

在开始锻炼时，要掌握正确的发音方式；控制音量，以自己耳朵能听见的音量为度；采用腹式呼吸、缩唇呼吸；每个动作要松柔舒缓；缓慢地增加运动次数，时间不宜过长。此外，锻炼总量要根据自身情况，逐渐进行增减。在锻炼的过程中会出现膝部微微酸痛，这属于正常情况。

第十三节　肩　　痛
Section 13　Shoulder Pain

1. Medical Theories Explained

Shoulder pain is a common symptom

1. 医说析疑

肩痛是我们大多数人

都会出现的一种症状,其中易引起肩痛的肩周炎是人们耳熟能详的存在。这也导致出现了肩部疼痛人们第一时间想到的就是肩周炎。人们对肩关节认识有限,常常把所有的肩关节疼痛都认为是肩周炎。其实"肩周炎"的发病率很低,绝大多数肩关节疼痛可能都不是"肩周炎",而可能是"肩袖损伤"。肩周炎多见于中老年人,多数患者呈慢性发病,一般年轻人不会得肩周炎,而更有可能是因为肩部过度使用或外伤引起的肩袖损伤。

肩关节疼痛,一定要明确病因。如果是肩袖损伤导致的肩关节疼痛,多运动反而可能会导致肩袖损伤的加重。如果是肩关节因为慢性疼痛逐渐出现活动度的情形,可以进行一些功能锻炼预防肩周软组织挛缩的加重,如做"手爬墙"的动作。导致肩关节疼痛的原因有很多,其中最常见的是由于肩峰撞击或老年退行性变导致的

experienced by many of us, with shoulder periarthritis being a well-known condition. This often leads to the assumption that shoulder periarthritis is the cause when people experience shoulder pain. People have limited awareness of shoulder joint diseases and often attribute all shoulder joint pain to shoulder periarthritis. However, the incidence of "shoulder periarthritis" is quite low, and the vast majority of shoulder joint pain may not be due to "shoulder periarthritis", but rather to "rotator cuff injuries". Shoulder periarthritis is more common in middle-aged and elderly individuals, with most patients experiencing a chronic course of the condition. Generally, young people are unlikely to develop shoulder periarthritis and are more likely to have rotator cuff injuries caused by overuse of the shoulder or trauma.

Shoulder joint pain need determining the cause. If the shoulder joint pain is due to a rotator cuff injury, excessive exercise may exacerbate the injury. If the shoulder joint pain is caused by chronic pain leading to a gradual decrease in mobility, some functional exercises can be done to prevent worsening of shoulder soft tissue contracture, such as the "wall climbing" exercise. There are many reasons for shoulder joint pain, but the most common cause is rotator cuff injury caused by shoulder impingement or age-related degenerative changes.

(1) Shoulder Periarthritis. Shoulder Periarthritis, commonly known as "frozen shoulder" or "adhesive capsulitis", refers to a tendon injury condition characterized primarily by shoulder joint pain and restricted movement due to extensive adhesions between the joint capsule and surrounding tissues. The condition typically involves progressively worsening shoulder pain, particularly at night, leading to widespread adhesions in soft tissues that restrict shoulder joint movement. As a result, shoulder joint mobility gradually diminishes. Once the pain and movement restriction reach a certain level, the condition tends to plateau, with pain gradually diminishing or disappearing and joint function gradually improving. However, in some cases, complete restoration to normal functional levels may not be achieved, leading to long-term shoulder joint pain and functional impairment. This condition is most common in individuals around the age of 50, with a higher incidence in females. It often occurs due to exposure to cold, overuse injuries, or prolonged immobilization of the shoulder joint. Without effective treatment, severe pain can disrupt sleep and may radiate to the neck, back, elbow, or hand. Severe restriction of shoulder joint movement can hinder daily activities such as combing hair, getting dressed, or washing the face. In

肩袖损伤。

（1）肩关节周围炎。简称肩周炎，俗称"漏肩风""冻结肩""五十肩"，是指关节囊与周围组织广泛粘连而引起以肩关节疼痛和活动功能障碍为主要特征的筋伤疾病。以肩周疼痛逐渐加重，夜间尤甚，逐渐引起软组织广泛性粘连，限制了肩关节活动，导致肩关节活动受限日益加重，当肩关节的疼痛与活动限制达到某种程度之后，就不再继续发展，并且疼痛逐渐减轻以致消失，关节的活动功能也逐渐恢复，但也有少部分不能完全恢复到正常功能水平，可有长期存在的肩关节疼痛和功能障碍。本病好发于50岁左右患者，女性发病率高于男性，多见于受凉、负重劳损及肩关节长时间不能自主活动引起。如得不到有效的治疗，剧烈的疼痛会影响睡眠，还可能会放射至颈背部、肘部或手部，肩关节活动严重受限的患者不能完成梳头、穿衣、洗脸等日常动作。病程长者还可出现肩臂不同程度的肌肉萎缩，尤以三角肌为明显。

（2）肩袖损伤。肩关节是上肢活动范围最大的关节，日常生活和工作中大部分的上肢活动都离不开它，如穿衣、梳头、洗脸、抬举重物等简单动作。肩袖损伤占肩关节疼痛疾病的 70%~80%。肩袖是肩关节周围的一组肌腱（由肩胛下肌、冈上肌、冈下肌及小圆肌组成），形似"袖口"，包裹肩关节的前方、上方及后方。肩袖的主要功能是为肩关节的活动提供力矩，满足肩关节外展、外旋、内旋等活动；还有就是给肩关节的稳定提供保证。

本病多见于重体力工作者或专业运动员。在日常生活中，中老年人群中比较常见到的是随着年龄的增长，肩袖组织会出现退行性变（即老化），易发生肩袖损伤。青年人群中比较常见于工作和生活中肩关节长期过度活动，以及健身锻炼过程中肌腱过度的拉伸负荷。还有就

chronic cases, muscle atrophy in the shoulder and arm may occur, particularly in the deltoid muscle.

(2) Rotator Cuff Injury. The shoulder joint is the joint with the widest range of motion in the upper limbs. Most activities of daily living and work involve it, such as dressing, combing hair, washing the face, and lifting heavy objects. Rotator cuff injuries account for 70% to 80% of shoulder joint pain conditions. The rotator cuff is a group of tendons (composed of the subscapularis, supraspinatus, infraspinatus, and teres minor muscles) surrounding the shoulder joint, resembling a "cuff", wrapping around the front, top, and back of the shoulder joint. The main function of the rotator cuff is to provide torque for the movements of the shoulder joint, such as abduction, external rotation, and internal rotation, and to ensure the stability of the shoulder joint.

This condition is more common in heavy manual laborers or professional athletes. In daily life, it is more common among middle-aged and elderly people as they age, as degenerative changes (aging) occur in the rotator cuff tissues, making them more prone to rotator cuff injuries. Among younger individuals, it is more common due to prolonged shoulder joint activity in work and daily life, as well as excessive stretching loads on the tendons during fitness exercises. Accidental falls where the palms or shoulders are impacted may also cause shoulder pain. Initially, when the injury is mild, the pain may not be obvious, but over time or with continued stretching exercises and excessive activity, the pain gradually worsens and can become severe, leading to serious rotator cuff injuries. The most common manifestation is restricted shoulder joint abduction (lifting the arm sideways from the body). Sometimes, there may be a sensation of the shoulder joint being locked or unable to continue moving, and all directions of shoulder joint movement may be restricted to varying degrees, with weakened strength and even inability to perform daily activities such as combing hair or raising the arms overhead. Typical pain characteristics include nighttime pain, pain when reaching behind the back, and a "painful arc". The acute phase treatment for rotator cuff injuries mainly involves immobilizing the shoulder joint. Once an acute injury occurs, immediate ice therapy should be applied to control possible aseptic inflammation or minor bleeding and swelling. During the recovery phase, restoring the mechanical balance of the rotator cuff and promoting the recovery of shoulder joint function are essential to meet daily life and exercise needs.

是生活中不小心摔倒时手掌撑地或肩部受到撞击后感到肩部疼痛，起初损伤较轻时疼痛不明显，随着时间推移或继续拉伸锻炼、过度活动后逐渐加重，疼痛可逐渐剧烈，容易引起严重肩袖损伤。最常表现为肩关节外展受限（从身体侧方上抬胳膊），有时可感觉到肩关节像被卡住、绞锁而不能继续活动，肩关节各个方向均有可能不同程度地受限，且有力量减弱，甚至无法进行梳头、手臂举过头顶等日常动作。患者典型疼痛特点为夜间痛、背手痛及"痛弧"。肩袖损伤的急性期治疗主要是肩关节制动，一旦发生急性损伤，应立即进行冰敷治疗，使可能出现的无菌性炎症或细微的出血、红肿得到控制。缓解期可以通过重建肩袖的力学平衡，促进肩关节功能的恢复，以满足生活和运动需要。

2. 防治方案

（1）改变生活中的不良习惯。注意肩部防寒保暖，尽量不要负重，不使肩关节过度疲劳。坚持合理的运动，加强肩部锻炼，增强肩部肌肉、韧带弹性。

（2）六字诀功法套路动作。反复练习整个套路动作，或侧重练习第一式"嘘"字诀，第四式"呬"字诀，第六式"嘻"字诀，每个字诀重复练习六遍，每天 2 次。

3. 习练秘诀

全身放松、精神集中、呼吸平稳，动作要松柔舒缓，配合呼吸、吐音协调自然地去练套路动作，注意每式动作的阴阳转换，促使身体肌肉关节的膨胀然后放松自然地转换。呼吸要求做到"匀、细、柔、长"，吸气时经鼻，每次吸气后不要忙于呼出，宜稍屏片刻，再徐徐呼出。

4. 注意事项

在开始锻炼时，要掌握正确的发音方式；控制

2. Prevention and Treatment Plan

(1) Changing Unhealthy Habits in Daily Life. Keeping the shoulders warm, avoid carrying heavy loads as much as possible, and prevent over-fatigue of the shoulder joints. Maintain a regular exercise by strengthening shoulder exercises, and enhancing the elasticity of shoulder muscles and ligaments.

(2) Liuzijue Routine Movements. Repeatedly practice the entire routine or focus on practicing the first posture "Xu", the fourth posture "Si", and the sixth posture "Xi". Repeat each posture six times, twice a day.

3. The Secret to Practice

Relax the whole body, concentrate the mind, and maintain steady breathing. Movements should be gentle and relaxed, coordinated with the breath and the pronunciation of the six sounds, naturally engaging in the practice routine. Pay attention to the transition of Yin and Yang in each posture, promoting the expansion and natural relaxation of muscles and joints. Breathing should be even, fine, gentle, and long. Inhale through the nose, and after each inhalation, avoid hasty exhalation; it's preferable to hold briefly before exhaling slowly.

4. Points to Note

When starting an exercise routine, it's important to master the correct pronunciation and control the volume, using the level audible to your own ears as a guide. Additionally, adopt abdominal breathing and pursed-lip breathing. Each movement should be gentle and relaxed, gradually increasing the number of repetitions and avoiding overly extended durations. Moreover, the overall exercise amount should be adjusted according to personal condition, gradually increasing or decreasing as needed. It's normal to experience slight soreness in the shoulders or knees in the course of practice.

音量，以自己耳朵能听见的音量为度；采用腹式呼吸、缩唇呼吸；每个动作要松柔舒缓；缓慢地增加运动次数，时间不宜过长。此外，锻炼总量要根据自身情况，逐渐进行增减。在锻炼的过程中会出现肩部、膝部微微酸痛，这属于正常情况。

第十四节　头　　痛
Section 14　Headache

1. Medical Theories Explained

Headache is one of the most common neurological disorders. The causes for the headache vary with complex manifesations. Some headaches are excruciatingly severe, others are mild and transient. Many people tend to endure headaches without seeking medical attention, assuming they will resolve them on their own. However, chronic or frequent headaches, especially those accompanied by fatigue, weakness, and neurological symptoms, may indicate an underlying condition that requires

1. 医说析疑

头痛是最常见的神经系统疾病之一。头痛的原因各异、症情复杂。有时头痛欲裂，有时很轻微，很多人觉得忍忍就过去了，没必要去看医生。如果慢性头痛或经常头痛，特别使人精神倦怠、神疲乏力、神经衰弱，患者通常对现有的治疗有抵抗或不耐受。临床上最常碰到的是紧张型头痛和药物过度使用型头痛，而不是我们常听到的偏头痛。

头痛分为原发性头痛和继发性头痛两大类型。头痛病因明确的，为继发性头痛，如脑膜炎、颅内肿瘤、脑外伤、药物过度使用及五官科等疾病引起的头痛；头痛找不到具体病因的，为原发性头痛，如紧张型头痛、偏头痛、丛集性头痛等。中医将头痛分为外感和内伤两大类。外感头痛主要病因是感受外邪诱发，以风邪为主。内伤头痛之病机多与肝、脾、肾三脏的功能失调有关，还有劳倦、饮食、房事不节及病后体虚等原因。头痛的表现多端，如药物过度使用型头痛，因长期过量使用止痛药物后出现的频繁发作的头痛，患者常有持续性头痛史，头痛几乎每天发生，且几乎持续整天时间，呈轻至中度钝痛，双侧或弥漫性疼痛，有时局限于额或枕部。紧张型头痛是非常普遍的，表现为两侧的持续钝痛，

medical intervention. The most common types of headaches encountered clinically are tension-type headaches and medication-overuse headaches, rather than migraines, which are frequently discussed.

Headaches are broadly categorized into primary and secondary types. Secondary headaches have identifiable causes, such as meningitis, intracranial tumors, head trauma, medication overuse, and disorders related to otolaryngology. Headaches without a specific underlying cause are classified as primary headaches, including tension-type headaches, migraines, and cluster headaches. In Traditional Chinese Medicine, headaches are classified into two categories: those caused by external pathogenic factors, primarily wind-cold or wind-heat invasion, and those resulting from internal imbalances, often related to dysfunction of the liver, spleen, and kidneys, as well as lifestyle factors like overwork, dietary irregularities, sexual excesses, and post-illness weakness. The manifestations of headaches are diverse. Medication-overuse headaches, for instance, occur frequently and persistently following prolonged and excessive use of analgesic medications. They typically present as daily or near-daily dull bilateral or diffuse headaches, lasting throughout the day. Tension-type headaches are prevalent and manifested by bilateral, dull, continuous pain lasting 30 minutes to several hours, typically without severely affecting daily activities. Associated symptoms may include pressure behind the eyes, tenderness of the head, face, and neck/shoulder muscles, as well as sensitivity to light and sound. Moreover, modern lifestyles, characterized by high work pressures, nocturnal smartphone use, and poor sleeping postures, contribute to an increased incidence of headaches, particularly migraines. Migraines typically manifest as severe throbbing pain on one side of the head, recurring over 3 days, often accompanied by sensitivity to light, sound, and odors, as well as nausea and vomiting. For many sufferers, migraines may persist throughout their lives.

2. Prevention and Treatment Plan

(1) Changing Unhealthy Habits in Daily Life. Rest and maintain a quiet environment with moderate lighting. Avoid excessive worrying, anger, and anxiety to reduce stress and maintain a cheerful mood. Adopt a healthy lifestyle by refraining from smoking and excessive alcohol consumption, avoiding staying up late, and steering clear of stimulating foods. Engage in regular and appropriate exercise to enhance physical fitness and strengthen the body's resistance to external pathogens.

(2) Liuzijue Routine Movements. Repeatedly practice the entire routine of

通常持续30分钟，甚至几个小时，但很少会影响日常生活。其他症状还包括眼后方压迫感，头面部和颈肩部的压痛，以及对光线和声音敏感等。另外，现在各行业的上班族，工作压力大，夜里玩手机睡不着，以及有些睡硬枕头，容易损伤颞肌引起偏头痛。偏头痛的性质主要为一侧剧烈的搏动性头痛，且反复发作，每次发作可能持续3天之久，患者可能会对光线、声音和气味很敏感，恶心和呕吐也很常见，对于很多人来说可能终身如此。

2. 防治方案

（1）改变生活中的不良习惯。注意休息，保持环境安静，光线不宜过强。避免忧思郁怒，减少焦虑和压力，保持心情愉悦。保持健康的生活方式，禁烟、戒酒，避免熬夜，避免刺激性饮食。坚持合理运动，增强体质，抵御外邪侵袭。

（2）六字诀功法套路动作。反复练习整个套路动作，或侧重练习第一式"嘘"字诀，第三式"呼"字诀，第五式"吹"字诀，每个字诀重复练习六遍，每天2次。

3. 习练秘诀

全身放松、精神集中、呼吸平稳，动作要松柔舒缓，配合呼吸、吐音协调自然地去练套路动作，注意每式动作的阴阳转换，促使身体肌肉关节的膨胀然后放松自然地转换。呼吸要求做到"匀、细、柔、长"，吸气时经鼻，每次吸气后不要忙于呼出，宜稍屏片刻，再徐徐呼出。按五行相生次序排列，"嘘"与肝相对应，肝属木，多锻炼"嘘"字功，具有疏通肝经、调畅气机、理气解郁的作用，可以改善肝阴不足、肝阳上亢而致头痛。运用腹式呼吸，会使气息流畅，产生柔和的内脏按摩作用，从而改善内脏功能。

4. 注意事项

在开始锻炼时，要掌

movements or focus on practicing the first posture "Xu", the third posture "Hu", and the fifth posture "Chui". Repeat each posture six times, twice a day.

3. The Secret to Practice

Relax the whole body, concentrate the mind, and maintain steady breathing. Perform the movements gently and smoothly, coordinating with the breath and vocalization naturally while practicing the routine. Pay attention to the transition of Yin and Yang in each posture, promoting the natural expansion and relaxation of muscles and joints. Regarding breathing, strive for even, fine, gentle, and long inhalations through the nose. After each inhalation, avoid hasty exhalation; instead, pause briefly and then exhale slowly. Following the sequence of the Five Elements, "Xu" corresponds to the Liver, which belongs to Wood. Therefore, practicing the "Xu" predominantly benefits the Liver, facilitating the smooth flow of Liver Qi and alleviating Qi stagnation and emotional constraint. This practice can help improve conditions such as Liver Yin deficiency or Liver Yang hyperactivity, which may lead to headaches. Employing abdominal breathing facilitates smooth airflow and gentle internal organs massage, enhancing visceral function.

4. Points to Note

When starting exercise, it's essential to

master correct pronunciation and control the volume, ensuring it's audible to your own ears. Utilize abdominal breathing and pursed-lip breathing techniques. Each movement should be gentle and relaxed, gradually increasing the number of repetitions while avoiding overly prolonged sessions. Additionally, adjust the total exercise amount gradually based on individual condition. It's normal to experience slight shoulder or knee discomfort in the course of practice.

握正确的发音方式；控制音量，以自己耳朵能听见的音量为度；采用腹式呼吸、缩唇呼吸；每个动作要松柔舒缓；缓慢地增加运动次数，时间不宜过长。此外，锻炼总量要根据自身情况，逐渐进行增减。在锻炼的过程中会出现肩部、膝部微微酸痛，这属于正常情况。

第十五节　慢性疲劳综合征
Section 15　Chronic Fatigue Syndrome

1. Medical Theories Explained

Chronic fatigue syndrome is characterized by persistent fatigue that cannot be explained by ordinary exertion or underlying medical conditions. The primary demographic has shifted from manual laborers to white-collar workers, particularly prevalent in industries such as internet technology, healthcare, banking, media, and education, showing a trend towards younger individuals. Many people nowadays experience a sense of exhaustion, reluctance to stand when they can sit, aversion to

1. 医说析疑

慢性疲劳综合征是一种慢性的、无法用一般劳累和疾病状况解释的疲劳症状。主要患者人群已从体力劳动者转向脑力劳动者，在互联网、医疗、银行、媒体、科教等行业的从业者中比较常见，并且呈现年轻化的趋势。现在很多人是能坐着不想站着、能躺着不想坐着、食欲不振、熬夜玩手机，还失眠多梦，有上不完的班，好像身体被掏空了，甚至躺着也总觉得累，累得感觉缓不过来，很可能是得了慢性疲劳综合征。根据疲劳产生的原因，可以分为生理性疲劳、心理性疲劳和病理性疲劳三类。生理性疲劳，也就是单纯的"累"了，多发生在体力劳动、运动之后或偶尔熬夜，一般好好休息后即可缓解。心理性疲劳，常见的原因是紧张、焦虑、抑郁等情绪因素导致的精力疲劳；病理性疲劳，比如贫血、睡眠障碍、甲状腺功能亢进或减退、骨关节疾病以及血脂血压异常等有明确病因的，都会让人容易感觉到累，只要从病根入手，对症治疗即可。慢性疲劳综合征的主要表现有注意力不集中、烦躁不安、神疲乏力、精神倦怠以及对工作和生活失去了热情，甚至会头昏气短、失眠、记忆力减退、抑郁等。

2. 防治方案

（1）改变生活中的不良习惯。保证充足睡眠，

sitting when they can lie down, loss of appetite, insomnia and vivid dreams, staying up late on their smartphones, an endless stream of work that leaves them feeling drained, exhausted though lying down. This could very well be chronic fatigue syndrome. Based on the causes of fatigue, it can be categorized into three types: physiological fatigue, psychological fatigue, and pathological fatigue. Physiological fatigue, simply feeling "tired", often occurs after physical exertion, exercise, or occasional late nights, and can typically be relieved with adequate rest. Psychological fatigue, commonly caused by stress, anxiety, depression, or other emotional factors leading to fatigue. Pathological fatigue, such as anemia, sleep disorders, hyperthyroidism or hypothyroidism, musculoskeletal disorders, and abnormal blood lipid or blood pressure levels, all have identifiable causes and can lead to feelings of exhaustion. Targeted treatment addressing the cause is necessary. The main manifestations of chronic fatigue syndrome include difficulty concentrating, irritability, mental fatigue, physical exhaustion, loss of enthusiasm for work and life, and symptoms like dizziness, shortness of breath, insomnia, memory impairment, and depression may also occur.

2. Prevention and Treatment Plan

(1) Changing Unhealthy Habits in Daily Life. Ensure an adequate amount of

sleep and avoid excessive fatigue and staying up late. Avoid dwelling on worries, anger, and reduce anxiety and stress. Maintain a healthy lifestyle by avoiding smoking and excessive alcohol consumption. Stick to a balanced diet, consume plenty of fruits and vegetables, stay hydrated, and avoid excessive intake of caffeine. Engage in regular exercise to increase the basal metabolic rate and enhance physical fitness.

(2) Liuzijue Routine Movements. Repeatedly practice the entire routine or focus on practicing the second posture "He". Repeat each posture six times, twice a day.

3. The Secret to Practice

Relax the whole body, focus the mind, maintain steady breathing. Movements should be gentle and relaxed, coordinated naturally with the breath and sound. Pay attention to the transformation of Yin and Yang in each posture, promoting the expansion and natural relaxation of muscles and joints. Breathing should be "even, fine, soft, and long", inhaling through the nose, and not rushing to exhale after each breath, but rather pausing briefly before slowly exhaling. Following the sequence of the Five Elements, "He" corresponds to the Heart, governing blood vessels and housing the spirit. Practicing the "He" posture can clear the Heart meridian, regulate the mind, and promote the circulation of blood within

生柔和的内脏按摩作用，从而改善肺脏、肾脏等功能。

4. 注意事项

在开始锻炼时，要掌握正确的发音方式；控制音量，以自己耳朵能听见的音量为度；采用腹式呼吸、缩唇呼吸；每个动作要松柔舒缓；缓慢地增加运动次数，时间不宜过长。此外，锻炼总量要根据自身情况，逐渐进行增减。在锻炼的过程中会出现肩部、膝部微微酸痛，这属于正常情况。

the Heart. Employing abdominal breathing facilitates smooth airflow and gentle internal organs massage, enhancing visceral function.

4. Points to Note

When starting to exercise, it's important to master correct pronunciation and control the volume, adjusting it to what you can comfortably hear. Additionally, adopt abdominal breathing and pursed-lip breathing. Each movement should be gentle and relaxed, gradually increasing the number of repetitions and avoiding overly long durations. Moreover, adjust the overall exercise intensity according to your own condition, gradually increasing or decreasing it as needed. It's normal to experience slight shoulder and knee soreness in the course of practice.

第十六节　便　秘
Section 16　Constipation

1. 医说析疑

便秘是一种常见的消化系统症状，是指排便的频率减少、排便不畅或大便干结难以排出的情况。尽管便秘通常不是严重问

1. Medical Theories Explained

Constipation is a common digestive symptom characterized by reduced frequency of bowel movements, difficulty passing stool, or dry and hard stools. While constipation is often not a serious problem, it can affect the quality of life for many people over the long term and may have negative impacts on health. Based on its causes, constipation can be classified into three main types: functional, organic, and drug-induced. Functional constipation, which is commonly encountered, is caused by dietary habits such as consuming overly refined foods, having excessive gastric heat, lack of exercise, high work pressure, or poor bowel habits. Organic constipation occurs due to certain diseases such as hemorrhoids, colorectal cancer, or diabetes. Drug-induced constipation refers to constipation caused by the use of calcium antagonists, antidepressants, or anticholinergic drugs. Nowadays, sedentary lifestyles, frequent consumption of takeout, and insufficient physical activity can result in deficiency of Yang Qi, leading to constipation. Therefore, it's important to engage in regular exercise to stimulate Yang Qi, promote colonic motility, and help restore physiological bowel rhythms, thus alleviating constipation.

2. Prevention and Treatment Plan

(1) Changing Unhealthy Habits in Daily Life. Maintain a regular lifestyle, quit smoking and drinking, avoid staying up late, and ensure an adequate amount of sleep. Stick to regular exercise to enhance gastrointestinal motility and increase the basal metabolic rate. Adjust dietary

题，但长期便秘影响着许多人的生活质量，可能会对健康产生负面影响。根据病因引起，便秘分为功能性、器质性和药物性三大类型。功能性便秘，也就是大家常遇到的一些因为饮食习惯而引起的便秘，如吃得太精细、体内胃火旺盛，或者缺乏运动、工作压力大、不良的排便习惯等。器质性便秘，则是由于某种疾病会出现便秘的情况，如痔疮、结直肠癌、糖尿病等。药物性便秘，是指使用钙拮抗剂、抗抑郁药、抗胆碱能药物等导致的便秘。现在的人们经常久坐不动、常吃外卖、缺乏运动。运动量小就会导致阳气不振，容易发生便秘。所以要多运动，可以激发阳气，刺激结肠蠕动，并帮助恢复结肠的生理节律的作用，缓解便秘。

2. 防治方案

（1）改变生活中的不良习惯。生活有规律，戒烟、戒酒，避免熬夜，保证充足的睡眠。坚持合理运动，增加胃肠蠕动功能，增加基础代谢率。调整饮食结构，饮食宜定时、适量，充足的水分摄入，多吃蔬菜和水果，增加膳食纤维。保持良好的排便习惯。

（2）六字诀功法套路动作。反复练习整个套路动作，或侧重练习第三式"呼"字诀，每个字诀重复练习六遍，每天2次。

3. 习练秘诀

全身放松、精神集中、呼吸平稳，动作要松柔舒缓，配合呼吸、吐音协调自然地去练套路动作，注意每式动作的阴阳转换，促使身体肌肉关节的膨胀然后放松自然地转换。呼吸要求做到"匀、细、柔、长"，吸气时经鼻，每次吸气后不要忙于呼出，宜稍屏片刻，再徐徐呼出。按五行相生次序排列，"呼"与脾相对应，脾属土、主运化，多锻炼"呼"字功，具有泻脾胃浊气、调理脾胃功能的作用，增强大肠传导功能。

4. 注意事项

在开始锻炼时，要掌

structure, consume meals at regular times and in appropriate amount, ensure sufficient intake of water, eat plenty of vegetables and fruits, and increase dietary fiber intake. Maintain good bowel habits.

(2) Liuzijue Routine Movements. Repeatedly practice the entire rountine movements, or focus on practicing the third posture "Hu", repeat six times, twice a day.

3. The Secret to Practice

Relax the whole body, concentrate the mind, maintain steady breathing, perform movements with softness and fluidity, coordinating with breath and sound, and practise the routine naturally. Pay attention to the transition of Yin and Yang in each posture, promoting the expansion and relaxation of muscles and joints in the body. Breathing should be "even, fine, gentle, and long", inhaling through the nose and not rushing to exhale immediately after each inhale; it is advisable to pause for a moment before exhaling slowly. Following the sequence of the Five Elements, "Hu" corresponds to the Spleen, which belongs to the Earth element and governs transformation. Practicing the "Hu" sound technique helps dispel turbid Qi from the Spleen and stomach, regulates their functions, and enhances the function of the large intestine.

4. Points to Note

When starting the exercises, it's

essential to master the correct pronunciation and control the volume, adjusting it to what you can hear with your own ears. Additionally, adopt abdominal breathing and pursed-lip breathing techniques. Each movement should be soft and gentle, gradually increasing the number of repetitions without overextending the duration. Furthermore, the overall exercise amount should be adjusted according to individual condition, gradually increasing or decreasing as needed. It's normal to experience slight shoulder or knee soreness in the course of practice.

握正确的发音方式；控制音量，以自己耳朵能听见的音量为度；采用腹式呼吸、缩唇呼吸；每个动作要松柔舒缓；缓慢地增加运动次数，时间不宜过长。此外，锻炼总量要根据自身情况，逐渐进行增减。在锻炼的过程中会出现肩部、膝部微微酸痛，这属于正常情况。

第十七节 肺 结 节
Section 17　Pulmonary Nodules

1. Medical Theories Explained

Pulmonary nodules are classically defined as round lesions with a diameter of ≤ 3 cm, detected on chest CT scans, exhibiting increased density. When there are two or more nodules, they are termed as multiple pulmonary nodules. Nodules with a diameter of ≤ 1 cm are referred to as small nodules, while those with a diameter < 5 mm are categorized as tiny nodules. Depending on the presence of ground-glass

1. 医说析疑

肺结节指在胸部 CT 检查中发现直径 ≤ 3cm、类圆形的、局灶性的、密度增高的病灶。2 个或者 2 个以上的结节称为多发性结节，结节直径 ≤ 1cm 称为小结节，直径 < 5mm 的结节称为微小结节。根据是否存在磨玻璃密度成分，肺结节包括纯磨玻璃结节、

混合磨玻璃结节以及实性结节，其中以混合磨玻璃结节最可能为恶性。越来越多的人在体检时或就诊其他疾病时发现肺结节。肺结节根据其生长性质，分为良性和恶性两种。肺结节的形成可能是多种疾病的表现，如受过外伤、得过肺炎或肺结核。另外其他多种多样的原因，比如年龄，长期主动或被动吸烟史，有恶性肿瘤疾病家族史及长期生活在雾霾、粉尘环境中等因素都有可能产生肺结节。

近年来由于新冠病毒的大流行及流感病毒的感染，人们咳嗽的频率增加了，病程变长了，引起了人们普遍的担心，逐渐开始重视关注肺结节了。其实，肺结节并不直接等于肺癌，大多数肺结节是良性的，随访是目前肺结节的主要防治手段。

2. 防治方案
（1）改变生活中的不良习惯。避免接触有毒有

opacity components, pulmonary nodules can be classified into pure ground-glass nodules, mixed ground-glass nodules, and solid nodules, with mixed ground-glass nodules being the most likely malignant. An increasing number of individuals discover pulmonary nodules during routine check-ups or while being treated for other conditions. Pulmonary nodules can be benign or malignant based on their growth characteristics. Various conditions, such as trauma, pneumonia, or tuberculosis, may lead to the formation of pulmonary nodules. Additionally, factors such as age, a history of active or passive smoking, a family history of malignant tumors, and prolonged exposure to pollution or dust, can contribute to their development.

In recent years, with the COVID-19 pandemic and the prevalence of influenza viruses, there has been an increase in cough frequency and prolonged illness duration, leading to widespread concerns and a growing awareness of pulmonary nodules. However, it's important to note that pulmonary nodules are not necessarily indicative of lung cancer. Most pulmonary nodules are benign, and regular follow-up is currently the primary means of prevention and management for pulmonary nodules.

2. Prevention and Treatment Plan
(1) Changing Unhealthy Habits in Daily Life. Avoid contact with toxic

substances, quit smoking and drinking. Avoid excessive worry, sadness, and anger to reduce anxiety and stress, maintaining a positive mindset. Maintain a healthy lifestyle, adhere to regular exercise, which helps improve cardiovascular and pulmonary function.

(2) Liuzijue Routine Movements. Practice the entire routine of movements, or focus on practicing the fourth posture "Si". Repeat each posture six times, twice a day.

3. The Secret to Practice

Relax the whole body, concentrate the mind, maintain steady breathing, perform movements gently and smoothly, coordinate with breathing and the pronunciation of "Si", and practice the routine naturally. Pay attention to the transformation of Yin and Yang in each posture, promoting the expansion and natural relaxation of muscles and joints in the body. Breathing should be "even, fine, gentle, and long", inhaling through the nose, and after each inhalation, it's advisable to pause briefly before exhaling slowly. According to the correspondence between organs and posture, "Si" corresponds to the Lungs. The Lungs govern respiration, control Water circulation, nourish the body's hundreds of vessels, and regulate the rhythm of the body. Practicing the "Si" posture helps clear the Lung meridian and regulate Lung function.

4. 注意事项

在开始锻炼时,要掌握正确的发音方式;控制音量,以自己耳朵能听见的音量为度;采用腹式呼吸、缩唇呼吸;每个动作要松柔舒缓;缓慢地增加运动次数,时间不宜过长。此外,锻炼总量要根据自身情况,逐渐进行增减。在锻炼的过程中会出现肩部、膝部微微酸痛,这属于正常情况。

4. Points to Note

When starting the exercise, it's important to master the correct pronunciation and control the volume, using the volume heard by your own ears as a reference. Additionally, adopt abdominal breathing and pursed-lip breathing techniques. Each movement should be performed gently and smoothly, gradually increasing the number of repetitions and avoiding overly long durations. Furthermore, the overall exercise intensity should be adjusted according to individual condition, gradually increasing or decreasing as needed. It's normal to experience slight shoulder or knee soreness in the course of practice.

第十八节 焦 虑
Section 18　Anxiety

1. 医说析疑

焦虑只是描述一种焦虑情绪状态。这种状态可以是适度的,也就是正常的,也可以是过度的,严重到疾病的程度就成为焦虑障碍了。在日常生活中,我们每一个人均会经历不同程度的焦虑、轻度的紧

1. Medical Theories Explained

Anxiety is simply a description of a state of anxious emotions. This state can be moderate, which is considered normal, or it can be excessive, reaching the level of a disorder known as anxiety disorders. In daily life, each of us experiences varying degrees of anxiety and mild tension. With the accelerating pace of work and increasing life pressures, more and more people are becoming concerned about psychological illnesses like "anxiety disorders". The causes of anxiety disorders can involve multiple factors including physiological, psychological, and social aspects. Physiologically, factors such as genetics, abnormal brain structure or function may form the basis for the onset of anxiety disorders. Psychologically, factors such as personality, thinking patterns, and stress coping abilities may affect the occurrence and development of anxiety disorders. Socially, factors such as life stress, psychological trauma, and tense interpersonal relationships can also serve as triggering factors for anxiety disorders. Clinical manifestations vary widely, mainly including excessive tension, fear, and anxiety, often accompanied by symptoms such as chest tightness, shortness of breath, palpitations, and sweating. These symptoms can significantly affect patients' daily lives and work, and even impact their overall physical and mental health.

In fact, anxiety often invisibly pervades our lives. Moderate anxiety can help mobilize bodily resources, unleash our full potential, and enhance our ability to cope with environmental pressures and handle work tasks. For example, moderate anxiety can sharpen our focus on tasks at hand, channel our energy towards problem-

张。随着工作节奏加快和生活压力的增大，越来越多的人开始关注"焦虑障碍"的心理疾病。其病因可涉及生理、心理和社会等多个方面。生理方面，如遗传、大脑结构或功能异常等因素可能是焦虑障碍的发病基础。心理方面，如性格、思维方式、抗压能力等可能影响焦虑障碍的发生和发展。社会方面，如生活压力、心理创伤、人际关系紧张等都有可能成为焦虑障碍的诱发因素。临床表现多种多样，主要包括过度紧张、害怕和恐惧等不安情绪，还可伴有胸闷、气短、心慌、出汗等症状。这些症状可能会严重影响患者的日常生活和工作甚至身心健康。

其实，焦虑常常无形地存在于我们的生活中。适度焦虑有利于调动身体资源，发挥最大的潜力，提高应对环境压力和处理工作的能力。例如，适度焦虑可以使注意力更加专注于正在做的事情，把精力更集中于要解决的问题，提升工作效率。当焦虑让自己感到不适，甚至感到痛苦，那就是过度了。过度焦虑会使注意力不容易集中、记忆力受到影响，使人容易感到疲惫，导致工作效率下降、容易出差错。短期过度焦虑可导致各种躯体症状、失眠障碍；长期过度焦虑易罹患高血压、冠心病、胃肠道疾病等疾病。

2. 防治方案

（1）改变生活中的不良习惯。正确对待各种事物，避免忧思郁怒，减轻压力。保持健康的生活方式，避免吸烟和过量饮酒，避免刺激性饮食。建立良好的社交关系，坚持合理运动。

（2）六字诀功法套路动作。练习整个套路动作，或者侧重反复练习第一式"嘘"字诀，第六式"嘻"字诀，每个字诀重复练习六遍，每天2次。

3. 习练秘诀

全身放松、精神集中、呼吸平稳，动作要松柔舒缓，配合呼吸、吐音协调自然地去练套路动作，注

solving, and boost work efficiency. However, when anxiety becomes distressing or even painful, it becomes excessive. Excessive anxiety can lead to difficulties in concentration, impaired memory, fatigue, decreased work efficiency, and increased likelihood of making mistakes. Short-term excessive anxiety can result in various physical symptoms and insomnia disorders, while long-term excessive anxiety may lead to conditions such as hypertension, coronary heart disease, and gastrointestinal disorders.

2. Prevention and Treatment Plan

(1) Changing Unhealthy Habits in Daily Life. Handle various situations appropriately, avoid excessive worry, sadness, and anger to reduce stress. Maintain a healthy lifestyle by avoiding smoking and excessive alcohol consumption, as well as overly stimulating diets. Foster good social relationships and commit to regular exercise.

(2) Liuzijue Routine Movements. Practice the entire routine of movements, or focus on practicing the first posture "Xu" and the sixth posture "Xi", repeat each posture six times each, twice a day.

3. The Secret to Practice

Relax the entire body, concentrate the mind, maintain steady breathing, perform movements gently and smoothly, coordinate with breathing, and naturally pronounce sounds while practicing the routine. Pay attention to the Yin-Yang transformation in each posture, promoting the expansion and natural relaxation of muscles and joints in the body. Breathing should be "even, fine, gentle, and long", inhaling through the nose, and after each inhalation, it's advisable to pause momentarily before exhaling slowly. According to the sequence of the Five Elements, "Xu" corresponds to the Liver, which belongs to the Wood element. Practicing the "Xu" posture helps clear the Liver meridian, regulate Qi flow, and relieve stagnation, improving Liver Qi stagnation syndrome and promoting a happy mood. Employing abdominal breathing facilitates smooth airflow and gentle internal organs massage, enhancing visceral function.

4. Points to Note

When starting exercise, it's important to master correct pronunciation and control volume, using the volume heard by your own ears as a guide. Additionally, adopt abdominal breathing and pursed-lip breathing techniques. Each movement should be gentle and relaxed, gradually increasing repetitions while avoiding overly long durations. Furthermore, adjust the overall exercise intensity according to personal condition, gradually increasing or decreasing as needed. It's normal to experience slight shoulder or knee soreness in the course of practice.

参考文献

[1] 吕立江.推拿功法学[M].北京：中国中医药出版社,2021:11.

[2] 梁·陶弘景,集.王家葵,校注.养性延命录校注[M].北京：中华书局,2014:199.

[3] 代金刚,曹洪欣,张明亮.《诸病源候论》呼吸吐纳法浅探[J].中医杂志,2016,57(3)：267–270.

[4] 张印生,韩学杰.孙思邈医学全书[M].北京：中国中医药出版社,2009:494.

[5] 高亮,赵玉坤,王宇新."六字诀"养生文化的起源、流变及其要义[J].体育与科学,2019,40(3)：80–85.

[6] 杨克新.健身气功全书[M].天津：天津科学技术出版社,2014：2–3.

[7] 苑沛然,孙志萍.2例新型冠状病毒肺炎患者应用"六字诀"呼吸操的护理[J].天津护理,2020,28(4)：431–433.

[8] 谢芳芳,管翀,成子己,等.传统功法对新冠肺炎呼吸系统和消化系统症状的防治[J].中医学报,2020,35(7)：1377–1382.

[9] 唐愿映,姬爱冬,邹缄,等."六字诀""呼"字功治疗孕期便秘临床观察[J].实用中医药杂志,2010,26(11):788–789.

[10] 陈锦秀,邓丽金.传统"六字诀呼吸操"对COPD稳定期患者的康复效果[J].中国康复医学杂志[J],2009,24(10)：944–945.

[11] 谢林艳,葛林阳,李涛,等.六字诀治疗慢性阻塞性肺疾病的价值及其应用[J].中华物理医学与康复杂志,2020,42(3)：285–288.

[12] 巨君芳,何迎春,李强,等.六字诀呼吸操联合穴位按摩改善老年COPD患者肺功能及生活质量的效果[J].中国现代医生,2019,57(27)：100–103.

[13] 贺晋芳."六字诀"呼吸法治疗COPD稳定期的疗效及对T淋巴细胞亚群的影响[D].北京：北京中医药大学,2019.

[14] 沈倩."六字诀"养生功法操对老年COPD稳定期（I级）患者社区干预的研究[J].中医临床研究,2017,9(23)：23–25.

[15] 陈红英,彭磊,范毕辉,等.健身"六字诀"结合益气活血法促进COPD稳定期患者肺康复的临床研究[J].河南中医,2016,36(5)：835–837.

[16] 樊雨倩,张聪,朱育萱,等.吐纳呼吸操联合穴位贴敷治疗

支气管哮喘慢性持续期临床观察 [J]. 安徽中医药大学学报，2021，40（3）：55–59.

[17] 涂人顺，张国玺. 健身气功·六字诀对中老年人身体形态、机能、素质和运动能力的影响 [C]. 北京：第六次全国中西医结合养生学与康复医学学术研讨会论文集，2009:26.

[18] 李敏，赖连花，赖渊杰，等. 嘘字诀用于急性期神经根型颈椎病镇痛的临床护理观察 [J]. 中国中医药现代远程教育，2016，14(15):49–50.

[19] 郑建寅，谢宁，王善祥，等. 慢性下腰痛患者呼吸肌功能评价及其相关分析 [J]. 颈腰痛杂志，1999，20（4）：269–270.

[20] 周国庆，姚新苗，李华，等. "六字诀"与腰椎核心稳定性训练的内在联系 [J]. 康复学报，2016，26(4):47–51.

[21] 王立红，张跃，白璧辉，等. 中医传统运动与骨质疏松症相关性研究现状 [J]. 中国骨质疏松杂志，2019，25(08)：1086–1091，1099.

[22] 涂人顺，陈仁波，黄林英，等. 传统健身方法（"六字诀"）对绝经期后女性内分泌水平的影响 [J]. 世界中西医结合杂志，2010，5(10):866–867.

[23] 赵芸溪，李翠华. 团队心理护理对抑郁症患者个人和社会功能的影响 [J]. 中西医结合护理（中英文），2017，3（4）：149–150.

[24] 高瑾. 六字诀对抑郁症患者抑郁、焦虑情绪的影响 [D]. 福州：福建中医药大学，2020.

郑重声明

高等教育出版社依法对本书享有专有出版权。任何未经许可的复制、销售行为均违反《中华人民共和国著作权法》，其行为人将承担相应的民事责任和行政责任；构成犯罪的，将被依法追究刑事责任。为了维护市场秩序，保护读者的合法权益，避免读者误用盗版书造成不良后果，我社将配合行政执法部门和司法机关对违法犯罪的单位和个人进行严厉打击。社会各界人士如发现上述侵权行为，希望及时举报，我社将奖励举报有功人员。

反盗版举报电话　（010）58581999　58582371

反盗版举报邮箱　dd@hep.com.cn

通信地址　北京市西城区德外大街 4 号　高等教育出版社知识产权与法律事务部

邮政编码　100120

读者意见反馈

为收集对教材的意见建议，进一步完善教材编写并做好服务工作，读者可将对本教材的意见建议通过如下渠道反馈至我社。

咨询电话　0086-10-58581350

反馈邮箱　xp@hep.com.cn

通信地址　北京市西城区德外大街 4 号

　　　　　高等教育出版社海外出版事业部（国际语言文化出版中心）

邮政编码　100120

防伪查询说明

用户购书后刮开封底防伪涂层，使用手机微信等软件扫描二维码，会跳转至防伪查询网页，获得所购图书详细信息。

防伪客服电话　（010）58582300

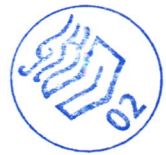